BioNanotechnology

BioNanotechnology

Elisabeth S. Papazoglou, Aravind Parthasarathy

www.morganclaypool.com

ISBN: 1598291386   paperback
ISBN: 9781598291384   paperback

ISBN: 1598291394   ebook
ISBN: 9781598291391   ebook

DOI: 10.2200/S00051ED1V01Y200610BME007

A Publication in the Morgan & Claypool Publishers' series
SYNTHESIS LECTURES ON BIOMEDICAL ENGINEERING #7

Lecture #7
Series Editor: John D. Enderle, University of Connecticut

Library of Congress Cataloging-in-Publication Data

Series ISSN: 1930-0328   print
Series ISSN: 1930-0336   electronic

First Edition
10 9 8 7 6 5 4 3 2 1

BioNanotechnology

Elisabeth S. Papazoglou, Aravind Parthasarathy
School of Biomedical Engineering
Drexel University

SYNTHESIS LECTURES ON BIOMEDICAL ENGINEERING #7

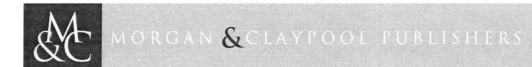
MORGAN & CLAYPOOL PUBLISHERS

ABSTRACT

This book aims to provide vital information about the growing field of bionanotechnology for undergraduate and graduate students, as well as working professionals in various fields. The fundamentals of nanotechnology are covered along with several specific bionanotechnology applications, including nanobioimaging and drug delivery which is a growing $100 billions industry. The uniqueness of the field has been brought out with unparalleled lucidity; a balance between important insight into the synthetic methods of preparing stable nano-structures and medical applications driven focus educates and informs the reader on the impact of this emerging field. Critical examination of potential threats followed by a current global outlook completes the discussion. In short, the book takes you through a journey from fundamentals to frontiers of bionanotechnology so that you can understand and make informed decisions on the impact of bionano on your career and business.

KEYWORDS

Bionanotechnology, Bionano initiatives, Bionano threats, Gold nanoparticles, Nano-bioimaging, Nano drug-delivery (or nano-vectors or targeted drug-delivery), Nano synthetics, and Bionanotoxicology, MRI, Titania nanoparticles, and Zinc nanoparticles.

Contents

Introduction

0.1 BIONANOTECHNOLOGY: *A Historical Perspective*

The first written concept of the possibility to manipulate matter at the nano-level was proposed by Richard Feynman who during his lecture "Room at the Bottom" discussed the use of atomic blocks to assemble at a molecular level [1, 2]. In this now famous quote, Feynman argues that, *"The principles of physics, as far as I can see, do not speak against the possibility of maneuvering things atom by atom. It is not an attempt to violate any laws; it is something, in principle, that can be done; but in practice, it has not been done because we are too big"* [2, 3]. In today's definitions, "nanotechnology is the understanding and control of matter at dimensions of roughly *1 to 100 nanometers*, where unique phenomena enable novel applications" [2–4].

The nanotechnology field was however really established by the work of Eric Drexler, Richard Smalley and in the bionanotechnology arena by Chad Mirkin.

a) Richard Smalley

Dr. Richard E. Smalley, a chemistry professor at Rice University, pioneered the field of nanotechnology and shared a Nobel Prize in 1996 for the development of bucky-balls, shown in Fig. 0.1. His contribution to nanotechnology is significant and the research team he established between Rice and the M.D. Anderson Cancer center has been a strong innovation force in the area of bionanotechnology.

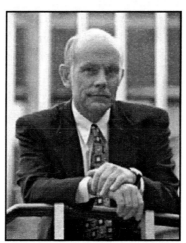

Dr. Richard E. Smalley—Nobel Laureate
(June 6, 1943–October 28, 2005)

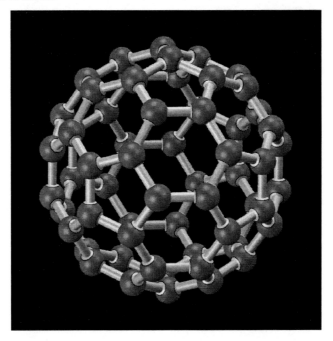

FIGURE 0.1: Fullerene (Bucky ball)—discovery by Dr. Richard Smalley

Smalley along with Robert Curl at Rice and Sir Harold Kroto at the University of Sussex discovered fullerenes, or bucky-balls, these unexpected spherical arrangements composed of 60 carbon atoms. Outside this fundamental, seminal contribution, Smalley's team continued with innovative contributions that impacted nanotechnology and its biomedical applications.

These include a practical way to produce large quantities of carbon nano tubes, a vital step in the commercial development of nanotechnology, and the founding of Carbon Nanotechnologies in 2000, to produce large quantities of nanotubes for research and commercialization.

b) Eric Drexler

K. Eric Drexler received his doctorate degree in *Molecular Nanotechnology* from MIT in 1991, the first degree of its kind. As a researcher, author, and policy advocate he has been one of the pioneers to focus on emerging technologies and their impact for the future.

He founded the Foresight Institute and presently serves as the Chief Technical Advisor of Nanorex, a company that develops software for the design and simulation of molecular machine systems. His thought provoking publications "Engines of Creation: The Coming Era of Nanotechnology," "Nanosystems: Molecular Machinery, Manufacturing, and Computation," and "Unbounding the Future: The Nanotechnology Revolution," made great impact by introducing the very topic of nanotechnology to many, and exposing an engineering approach

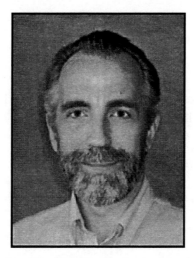

Dr. Eric Drexler *(April 25, 1955-)*

to nanotechnology and nanosystems [5–6]. In *Chapter 7*, we will see a summary of ideas exchanged between Richard Smalley and Eric Drexler on the feasibility and scope of "molecular assemblers" with regard to future [6].

c) Chad Mirkin

Chad A. Mirkin is presently a Professor in the Department of Chemistry and Institute for Nanotechnology at Northwestern University, and has been a pioneer in chemical modifications of nanosystems leading to breakthrough contributions to bionanotechnology.

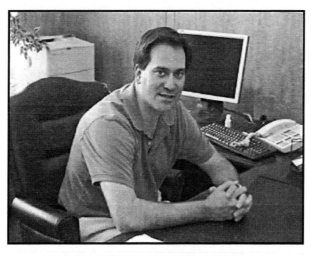

Dr. Chad Mirkin *(November 23, 1963-)*

His research work focusing on new ligand design, self-assembled monolayers, design of molecule-based electronic devices, nanolithography, nanoparticles, and DNA-directed materials synthesis provided the foundation for bionanotechnology research in many diverse application areas [7–18].

A most insightful quote of **Chad Mirkin** explains the need to open our minds and change our attitude as we embark on learning this new field: *"At the nano level atoms do not belong to any field of science."* In a very elegant way, this conveys the extreme diversity and uniqueness of nanotechnology, while stressing the preparation required by those aspiring to contribute to it. Our goal in this short book is to expose the reader in a methodical way to the necessary concepts and key advances of the field so as to enable further study of the subject or an informed decision involving use of bionanotechnology.

0.2   NANOTECHNOLOGY AND BIONANOTECHNOLOGY

In an effort to define the borders of this new and emerging discipline the National Nanotechnology Institute (NNI) proposed the limitation that truly "nanotechnology is the understanding and control of matter at dimensions of roughly 1 to 100 nm, where unique phenomena enable novel applications" [4]. As length scale is a continuum, a seeming fuzziness exists in the transition from the micrometer to the nanometer scale. For example, are structures of 800 nm (0.8 microns) true nanostructures or not?

According to the NNI definition, any structure less than 100 nm is a true nanostructure and unique phenomena are expected at that scale [4]. By the same approach however, if novel phenomena are exhibited by a structure at 200 nm this is a nanotechnology enabled material and as such is the realm of study in nanotechnology.

Nanotechnology is defined as, engineering and manufacturing at nanometer scales, with atomic precision. The term is interchangeable with "molecular nanotechnology" [1].

Bionanotechnology is a subset of nanotechnology where the biological world provides the inspiration and/or the end goal. It is defined as atom-level engineering and manufacturing using biological precedence for guidance (Nano-Biomimetics) or traditional nanotechnology applied to biological and biomedical needs [1].

In order to gain a feeling of the relative size of a nanometer, let us compare some everyday objects with some biological basic blocks using a nano-ruler. Table 0.1 summarizes several such examples including Qd, Micelles, glucose, nanoparticles, and hemoglobin. For instance, the thickness of human hair is 50,000 nm, while the size of a glucose molecule is less than 1 nm [19]. It is remarkable that a molecule 50,000 times smaller in size than one strand of human hair provides energy for our metabolic activities. Table 0.1 compares entities of bionanotechnology with matters of daily life so as to give a lucid picture of what it takes to be nano and to feel how small they are. Other examples of nano entities could be found elsewhere [19].

TABLE 0.1: Comparison of Nanoparticles with Matter of Macro World

1.	Glucose molecule diameter: 1 nm	Thickness of human hair 0.050 mm	Thickness of human hair 0.050 mm	A man of 8.3 feet height
	1:	50,000	1:	50,000
2.	Gold nanoparticle of diameter: 8 nm	Apple of diameter: 8 cm	Apple of diameter 8 cm	65% of diameter of earth 0.65 *12,576 km = 8,170 km
	1:	10,000,000	1:	10,000,000
3.	Micelle diameter: 13 nm	Soap bubble 1.3 cm	Soap bubble of 1.3 cm	Diameter of earth 12,576 km
	1:	10,000,000	1:	10,000,000
4.	Quantum dot diameter: 20 nm	Diameter of a cent 1.9 cm	Diameter of a cent 1.9 cm	55% of diameter of moon 1,9050 km
	1:	10,000,000	1:	10,000,000
5.	Hemoglobin diameter: 6.5 nm	Riffle bullet of diameter: 6.5 mm	Riffle bullet of diameter: 6.5 mm	A land of diameter 6.5 km (three times as big as Vatican City)
	1:	1,000,000	1:	1,000,000

0.3 NOTABLE NANOIMAGES IN BIONANOTECHNOLOGY
0.3.1 AFM-Qd

Fig. 0.2 is an image of quantum dots (QDs) obtained from the atomic force microscope (AFM) which will be discussed in detail in *Chapter 3*. The AFM is a form of microscope having the ability to image nano-sized objects. The imaging of nano-sized objects is facilitated via mechanical interaction of a very sensitive tip (which is the probe of the microscope) with the sample. The quantum dots or QDs are semiconductor particles of smaller diameters ranging between 2- and 10 nm.

Their small size, sharp optical features, and excellent fluorescence make them an ideal candidate for biological imaging applications [20]. Fig. 0.2 shows an AFM image of quantum dots made of InAs imaged at 1 μm × 1 μm [21].

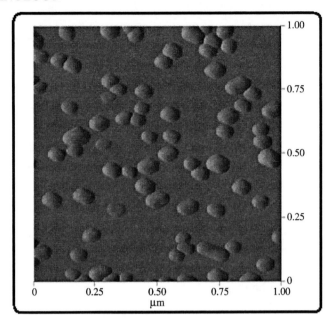

FIGURE 0.2: AFM image of quantum dots

0.3.2   Nano-drug Delivery Chip

Fig. 0.3 is an image of the front and back views of a drug delivery microchip made of silicon and coated with gold, with a U.S. dime (10 cents). The chip in the picture consists of 34 nano-sized wells each of which is capable of housing 24 nl (nano liters) of drug. It is possible to make at least 400 wells or even 1000 or more in these chips which are very inexpensive, costing less than $20 [22, 23].

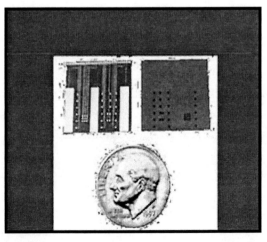

FIGURE 0.3: Drug delivery microchip

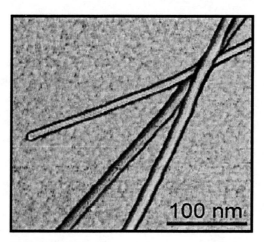

FIGURE 0.4: SWNT ropes with SWNT probe

0.3.3 Atomic Force Microscopy Image (AFM) of SWNT

Fig. 0.4 shows the AFM image of single wall carbon nanotube **(SWNT)** bundles obtained with a SWNT probe (tip), by using a phase contrast technique [24].

0.3.4 Scanning Electron Microscopy Image (SEM) of SWNT

Fig. 0.5 shows the scanning force micrograph of "crop circle" of SWNT. The circle has an apparent height of 1.0–1.2 nm and a width of 4–8 nm. The actual tube height is close to 1.5 nm (typical of SWNT) [25].

The carbon nanotubes (CNT) will be discussed in detail, later in *Chapter 5*.

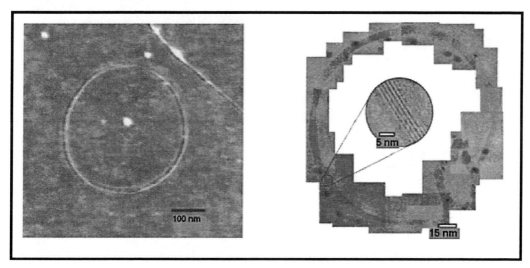

FIGURE 0.5: SEM images of CNT

0.4   OPPORTUNITIES AND CHALLENGES OF BIONANOTECHNOLOGY

The size of one to several nanometers is of central importance to life, justifying the term "nature's yard stick" for this dimension. The size of cellular organelles and other interesting objects with regard to bionanotechnology is summarized in the following graph, Fig. 0.6.

It is then easy to understand that interacting, controlling, and altering cellular and subcellular organelles, protein molecules, receptors, and cytokines can be achieved best with structures at the same size level as the biomolecular components of interest. Already capabilities made possible by fluorescent semiconductor nanoparticles, known as quantum dots, allowed dynamic angiography in capillaries hundreds of micrometers below the skin of living mice. This corresponds to about twice the depth of conventional angiographic materials and has been obtained with one-fifth of the irradiation power [26]. The development of hyperthermia nano agents for cancer therapy is underway and could impact patients in the next 2–5 years [27], while transparent sun screens sensing the amount of damage to skin are the next generation products in the sun protection industry [26, 28].

An example of advances in other nanotechnology fields that impact bionanotechnology is the successful development of nanotube-based fibers requiring three times the energy-to-break of the strongest silk fibers and 15 times that of Kevlar fiber; such fibers are further functionalized to detect toxic agents and deliver protection and warning to the user [29]. Examples of successful water decontamination where iron particles can remove up to 96% of trichloroethylene from groundwater are another application of bionanotechnology where environmental remediation can be accomplished [18].

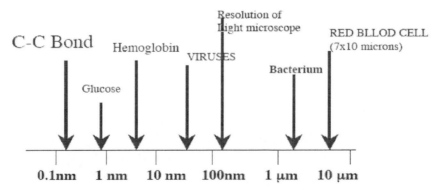

FIGURE 0.6: Various nano-sized entities in bionanotechnology [Courtesy of Dr. Papazoglou, Drexel University]

Disease treatment is reaching a turning point, with the emerging fields of molecular based medicine and personalized medicine. A cellular level control is not possible without nanotechnology as the key enabling technology. We can look forward to clinicians diagnosing diseases much faster with higher sensitivity and specificity. The possibilities of developing multifunctional nano-devices are attracting more attention [28]. This creates a collaborative effort for different fields to come together and collectively advance knowledge in solving a problem. Molecular understanding of cellular function in health and disease is augmented by nano-tools, while disease treatment is also impacted by the same methods. The distinctions of basic and applied science merge as they synergize each other to improve human health.

An example of a persistent difficult problem to understand in detail from *nature* involves the dynamics of self-assembly [30, 31]. Bionanotechnology could allow us to synthesize biomimetic nanostructures [30] to control and model the self-assembly process. This would be an area where nanotechnology helps augment our basic biological understanding [31].

The greatest challenge of bionanotechnology today is understanding the long-term impact on human health and the environment of structures we cannot see even with the most sophisticated optical microscopes and structures that can interact with the basic components of life. A scientific approach of utmost rigor is required to reveal interactions of nanostructures that may be affecting human health [23, 26, 28, 32].

0.5 GROWTH POTENTIAL OF NANOTECHNOLOGY AND RELATED EXPENDITURES

The opportunity for nanotechnology to revolutionize diverse technical areas has been well understood. It is not easy to estimate the expenditures for bionanotechnology from the pooled nanotechnology investment.

Conservative estimates place the bionanotechnology portion to at least 50% of nanotechnology dollars spent, while breakthroughs and advances in the general nanotechnology field benefit bionanotechnology directly or indirectly. Table 0.2 provides a yearly summary of the US national level expenditure incurred in the field of nanotechnology [33, 34].

The projection of expenditures shows a drastic increase with forecasts anticipating an astounding $1 Trillion by the year 2015 [35]. The 21st Century Nanotechnology Research and Development act [35] of the US senate enables and encourages such high level of expenditures to ensure the competitiveness of the US workforce in the global environment [35–38].

YEAR	ANNUAL BUDGET USD IN MILLIONS
TABLE 0.2: Yearly US Nanotechnology Expenditure during 1997–2015	
1997	116
1998	190
1999	255
2000	270
2001	465
2002	697
2003	862
2004	961
2005	1,200
2006	1,302.5
2007	1,278.3*
2015	1,000,000
NOTE: Year 2007* is subjective to changes.	

It can confidently, be stated that:

1. Nanotechnology is still in its infancy and has an almost unpredictable growth, which seems steady and increasing.

2. The field has excellent potential to consume more resources attracting further investment.

The following graph in Fig. 0.7 (adapted from Roco, M.C. and NNI budget for 2007) shows the yearly expenditures incurred in nanotechnology research [33, 34].

A global comparison of the annual expenditure in nanotech research reveals a similar trend as observed in the United States. Fig. 0.7 charts a comparison of US annual expenditures in nanotechnology versus Western Europe, Japan, and Others [39]. May it be global or in the United States, the research initiatives and expenditure in nanotechnology are steadily increasing.

The growth and the present trend in nanotechnology as well as bionanotechnology are quite promising and booming. A detailed insight into international Bionanotechnological initiatives and funding will be dealt in detail in *Chapter 7*.

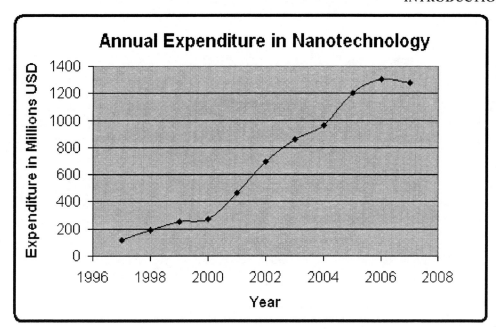

FIGURE 0.7: Annual Research Expenditure in Nanotechnology in the US

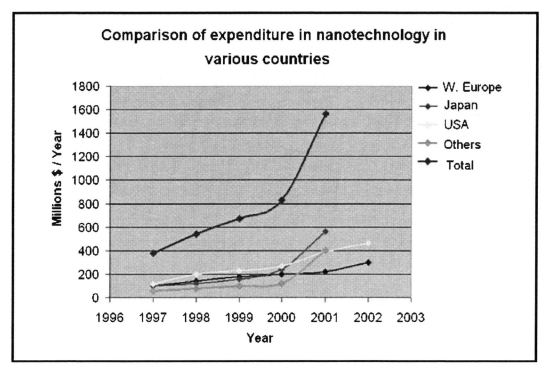

FIGURE 0.8: Annual nanotechnology expenditure—a global outlook (Adapted from ref. [39])

REFERENCES

[1] D. S. Goodsell, *Bionanotechnology: Lessons from Nature*. Willey-Less, 2004, pp. 1–8 (311), New Jersey, USA.

[2] R. Feynman, *There's Plenty of Room at the Bottom*. The Vega Science Trust, December 29th 1959, The American Physical Society at CalTech, California.

[3] R. Feynman, *There's Plenty of Room at the Bottom*. 1959 [cited 2006 10/02/2006]; [Transcript]. Available from: `http://www.zyvex.com/nanotech/feynman.html` [A website based from Georgia].

[4] (NNI), N.N.i. *Nanotechnology: What is Nanotechnology?* 2000 [cited 2006 10/2/2006]; Available from: `http://www.nano.gov/html/facts/whatIsNano.html` [It is a webpage, place of publication unkonwn].

[5] E. K. Drexler, *Nanotechnology Essays: Revolutionizing the Future of Technology [EurekAlert! Incontext]*. 2006 [cited 2006 10/02/2006]; Available from: http://www.eurekalert.org/context.php?context=nano&show=essays [Washington DC, USA].

[6] R. Baum, "Nanotechnology: Drexler and Smallye make the case for and against molecular assemblers," *Chem. Eng. News*, vol. **81**, pp. 37–42, 2003.

[7] M. Covington, et al., "Observation of surface-induced broken time-reversal symmetry in YBa2Cu3O7 tunnel junctions," *Phys. Rev. Lett.*, vol. **79**, pp. 277–280, 1997.

[8] R. Elghanian, et al., "Selective colorimetric detection of polynucleotides based on the distance-dependent optical properties of gold nanoparticles" *Science*, vol. **277**, pp. 1078–1080, 1997.

[9] B. J. Holliday, and M.C. A., "Strategies for the construction of supramolecular compounds through coordination chemistry," *Angew. Chem., Int. Ed.*, vol. **40**, pp. 2022–2043, 2001.

[10] R. Jin, et al., "Photo-induced conversion of silver nanospheres to nanoprisms" *Science*, vol. **294**, pp. 1901–1903, 2001.

[11] C. A. Mirkin, et al., A DNA-based method for rationally assembling nanoparticles into macroscopic materials. *Nature*, vol. **382**, pp. 607–609, 1996.

[12] S. J. Park, T. A. Taton, and C. A. Mirkin, Array-based electrical detection of DNA using nanoparticle probes. *Science*, **295**, pp. 1503–1506, 2002.

[13] R. D. Piner, et al., Dip pen nanolithography. *Science*, vol. **283**): pp. 661–663, 1999.

[14] J. J. Storhoff, et al., One-Pot Colorimetric Differentiation of Polynucleotides with Single base imperfections using gold nanoparticle probes. *J. Am. Chem. Soc.*, vol. **120**(9), pp. 1959–1964, 1998.

[15] J. J. Storhoff, and C. A. Mirkin, Programmed materials synthesis with DNA. *Chem. Rev.*, vol. **99**, pp. 1849–1862, 1999.

[16] J. J. Storhoff, R. C. Mucic, and C. A. Mirkin, Strategies for organizing nanoparticles into aggregate structures and functional materials. *J. Clust. Sci.*, vol. **8**, pp. 179–216, 1997.

[17] T. A. Taton, C. A. Mirkin, and R. L. Letsinger, Scanometric DNA array detection with nanoparticle probes. *Science*, vol. **289**, pp. 1757–1760, 2000.

[18] W.-X. Zhang, Nanoscale iron particles for environmental remediation: an overview. *J. Nanopart. Res.*, vol. **5**(3-4), pp. 323–332, 2003.

[19] C. Bruce, Nanotechnology: molecular speculations on global abundance, B. C. Crandall, Ed., MIT Press, 1996, pp. 1–5 (226) [Cambridge, MA, USA].

[20] A. Smith, et al., Engineering luminescent quantum dots for invivo molecular and cellular imaging. *Ann. Biomed. Eng.*, vol. **34**(1): pp. 3–14, 2006.

[21] S. Barik, H. H. Tan, and C. Jagadish, Comparison of InAs quantum dots grown on GaInAsP and InP. *Nanotechnology*, vol. **17**, pp. 1867–1870, 2006.

[22] R. Langer, and N. A. Peppas, Advances in biomaterials, drug delivery, and bionanotechnology. *Bioeng., Food, Natural Prod.—AIChE*, vol. **49**(12), pp. 2090–3006, 2003.

[23] E. A. Thomson, *Microchip Stores, Releases Chemicals for Many Uses.* 1999 [cited 2006 10/02/1006]; Available from: http://web.mit.edu/newsoffice/1999/chip-0203.html.

[24] F. Nano, *SWNT Ropes with SWNT Probe.* [Bitmap Image] 2005 [cited 2006 10/02/2006]; Available from: http://www.firstnano.com/applications.html# .

[25] J. Liu, et al., Fullerene crop circles. *Nature*, vol. **385**, pp. 780–781, 1997.

[26] T. W. Foundation, The Whitaker Foundation 2004 Annual Report: Biomedical Engineering and the Medical Applications of Nanotechnology, The Whitaker Foundation, pp. 1–48, 2004.

[27] D. Misirlis, "Development of a novel drug delivery system based on polymeric, thermoresponsive, hydrogel nanoparticles," in *Institute of Integrated Biosciences*, École Polytechnique Fédérale De Lausanne, pp. 1–149, 2005.

[28] W. C. W. Chan, Bionanotechnology progress and advances. Biol. Blood Marrow Transplant., vol. **12**, pp. 87–91, 2006.

[29] C. Q. Sun, et al., Dimension, strength, and chemical and thermal stability of a single C-C bond in carbon nanotubes. *J. Phys. Chem. B*, vol. **107**, pp. 7544–7546, 2003.

[30] Z. Ökten, et al., Myosin VI walks hand-over-hand along actin. *Nat. Struct. Mol. Biol.* vol. **11**, pp. 884–887, 2004.

[31] P. D. Vogel, Nature's design of nanomotors. *Eur. J. Pharm. Biopharm.*, vol. **60**, pp. 267–277, 2005.

[32] I. L. Medintz, et al., Self-assembled nanoscale biosensors based on quantum dot FRET donors. *Nat. Mater.*, vol. **2**, pp. 630–638, 2003.

[33] (NNI), N.N.I., *NNI Annual Budget for 2007: Supplement to the President's 2007 Budget*, N.S.a.T.C. (NSTC), NNI, pp. 1–76, 2006.

[34] M. C. Roco, The US National Nanotechnology Initiative after 3 years (2001–2003). *J. Nanopart. Res.*, vol. **6**, pp. 1–10, 2004.

[35] US, G., *The 21st Century National Nanotechnology Research and Development Act.* pp. 1–2, 2004.

[36] (NSTC), N.S.a.T.C., *National Nanotechnology Initiative and a Global Perspective. "Small Wonders", Exploring the Vast Potential of Nanoscience,* pp. 1–8, 2002.

[37] (WTEC), W.T.E.C., *Nanostructure Science and Technology: R&D Status and Trends in Nanoparticles, Nanostructured Materials, and Nanodevices. [Chapter 12],* R.S.H.-P. Williams and G.D.U. Stucky, Eds., pp. 181–201 1998.

[38] R. Lux, *The Nanotech Report 2004.* 2004 [cited; Available from: http://www.nanoxchange. com/NewsFinancial.asp?ID=264.

[39] M. C. Roco, *National Nanotechnology Initiative and a Global Perspective. "Small Wonders", Exploring the Vast Potential of Nanoscience,* 2002, National Science and Technology Council (NSTC), Nanoscience, Engineering and Technology (NSET), pp. 1–8.

CHAPTER 1

The Significance of Nano Domain

1.1 LIMITATIONS OF MICRON SIZE

In biomedical applications such as drug delivery and imaging, size plays a significant role in the efficacy and success of the treatment. Macro size has notable draw-backs when compared to nano-size with regard to biological applications, due to the size of cellular and subcellular compartments. For instance, conventional micron-size drug delivery techniques in cancer therapy suffer from inefficacy of delivery, inadequate targeting, toxic effects on healthy tissues, and impaired transport to tumor sites.

Earlier in drug delivery applications, different modes of administering the drug such as oral, nasal, transdermal, intra venal, and others were adapted. Oral and nasal deliveries exhibit high drug levels in blood and have poor release profiles; aerosol design is complex and problematic with regard to loading issues, while transdermal delivery lacks targeting and causes damage to healthy cells too [1]. These challenges led to the development of "targeted drug delivery" as a way to overcome the delivery issues. However, micron sized (μm) delivery vehicles cannot traverse in a passive fashion through cells and cell pores, and this also includes tumor cells with pore sizes as big as 380–780 nm. As a result, the ideal system for biological applications would be a targeted nano-delivery system [2–4].

1.2 NEED FOR NANO-SIZE—SURFACE VOLUME RATIO SIGNIFICANCE

For smaller/finer particles the area occupied by a unit volume of the nano-particles is higher than that occupied by the same volume of micron sized particle; therefore the number of particles available per square unit of area in a nano system is very much higher than a bigger (micron) sized system. The surface area when divided by the volume of the sample gives the *surface area to volume ratio*; this is a very significant factor which determines the extent of activity of a nanoparticulate system [5]. In a sample of NPs, the greater the surface to volume ratio the greater is its activity (catalytic or drug delivery related) [6]. This has been demonstrated with nano-particles of gold, titania, zinc oxide, palladium [7].

1.3 SIGNIFICANCE AND KEY FEATURES OF NANO-SIZE

The world of nano conflicts with the macro world in almost every functionality. The nano-world is immune to laws of gravity and inertia unlike the macro world. Nano-machines and nano-particles may appear "weird" owing to utmost disobedience to Newtonian Physics of inertia and gravity. For instance, the bacterial model discussed by Purcell is a classic example of the nano (micro as well) world's disobedience to the laws of inertia. The bacterial cell uses a flagellum to swim in water and is able to come to an abrupt halt without any observed inertia [8]. Our expectation to see an inertial effect before the stop, i.e., to see it move further and then stop is not observed. This puzzle is solved when we consider that inertial effects are negligible at that size and not observable by us. The contribution of inertial effects to the bacterium's motion before the halt is less than the diameter of an atom (in Angstroms) [8].

Another fascinating aspect is the negligible impact of gravity on nano-particles (NP). In the nano-world, particle–particle attractions/repulsions are more prominent than gravitational forces. For instance, water droplets hanging down from the ceiling are an excellent example of particle–particle attraction being far greater than the pull of gravity in small sized systems. Having said about the failure of classical physics in governing the nanosystems, it is much with the phenomenon associated with the quantum world that better dictate the performance of nanoparticulate systems.

A nanoparticulate system may be sensitive to its environmental conditions such as temperature, visible light, ultraviolet (UV), infrared (IR), etc. depending on its own physical and chemical properties. Hess and Mikhailov put forth that, any two molecules "within a μm sized cell meet each other every second." Thermal energy (heat) provides a driving force, by increasing the diffusion and the system's physiochemical interactions [8]. There are also some general factors that interact with most of the nanoparticulate systems; this includes pH, and surface charge (forces of attraction/repulsion), and vibration forces, centrifugation, stirring etc. can easily and effectively impact a nanoparticulate system. A notable and important aspect of the NPs system is that of atomic granularity. The system is granular at the atomic dimensions; one cannot expect smooth surfaces or interfaces between different particles. The atom–atom interaction determines the NP's shape, size, geometry, and orientation. All the above-mentioned features greatly contribute to the "self-assembly" property of certain nanoparticulate systems, mostly observed in proteins and nature's biomachines [9, 10].

Measurements and characterization of NP systems are crucial processes during which one has to pay attention to bring the system to a complete rest. This is done to settle down the random Brownian motion which is observed in aqueous suspended NP systems. It is notable that many of the NP systems of interest to bionanotechnological applications are suspended in an aqueous phase in order to study its viability in aqueous medium; this is because, the cells in the human body have vast aqueous medium that the NP system will have to interact with [8].

As mentioned earlier, the laws of quantum mechanics govern the interaction of NP with their environment. Usually, in a system of NPs, the covalent bond holds intact one NP to the other, defining the particles' geometry and shape. Steric hindrance, electrostatic interaction, and hydrogen bonds also influence particle–particle interactions to a certain extent. Thus a system of NP under study should encompass all of the above-mentioned factors in order to understand and model the system.

1.4   DERIVATION OF BOHR'S ATOMIC RADIUS OF A HYDROGEN ATOM

The failure of classical physics to explain the properties of matter at the atomic scale led to the evolution of quantum mechanics. Fundamental concepts of quantum mechanics were developed by Neils Bohr who put forth in 1913 that in a free atom, electrons occupy discrete energy states associated with shells or orbits in an atom [11].

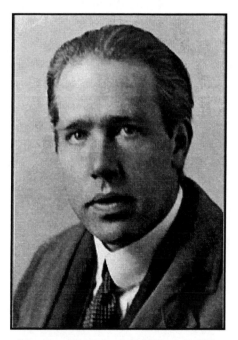

Neils Bohr 1885-1962
Noble Laureate - Physicist

Depending on the excitation energy electrons can jump from one energy level to the other. They later return to their ground state which is their most stable state.

Neils Bohr modeled and predicted the energy levels in a hydrogen atom which is popularly referred to as the Bohr's atomic model. This model serves as a corner stone for quantum theory which is able to answer various puzzles in physics with accuracy and precision that classical wave theory had not been able to resolve. Bohr's model is arguably the simplest and most realistic model of quantum mechanics [11].

Combining the energy of the classical electron orbit with the quantization of angular momentum, the Bohr approach yields expressions for the electron orbit radii and energies [11].

To arrive at the Bohr's radii of a hydrogen atom consider an electron of mass m present in an orbit of radius r with respect to the nuclei.

$$\text{Kinetic energy of electron} = \frac{mv^2}{2}$$

Angular momentum of the electron with respect to the nuclei

$$L = mvr \sin \theta$$

But $\theta = 90°$ for a circular orbit, so Sin 90 = 1.

Therefore angular momentum of the electron

$$L = mvr \tag{1.1}$$

Kinetic energy expressed as angular momentum

$$\frac{(mvr)^2}{2mr^2} \tag{1.2}$$

(this is same as $\frac{mv^2}{2} \frac{mv^2}{2}$).

According to DeBroglie's equation of wavelength,

$$\lambda = \frac{h}{p}$$

where

λ = wavelength in meters (m)

h = Planck's constant = 6.626×10^{-34} JouleSec. = 4.136×10^{-15} eV.Sec;

p = momentum $\dfrac{\text{kg.m}}{\text{Sec.}}$ = mass $\times$ velocity = mv.

Therefore

$$\lambda = \frac{h}{mv} \tag{1.3}$$

According to the standing wave condition, the circumference of an orbit of a particle (electron) is equal to the whole number times the associated wavelength.

$$\text{Circumference} = 2\pi r = n\lambda_n \quad \text{Or} \quad r = \frac{n\lambda}{2\pi} \tag{1.4}$$

where r is the radius of the orbit, n is the whole number of the associated orbit (nth orbit from the nuclei), and λ_n refers to the wavelength of the nth orbit.

By putting (1.3) in (1.1) we get ......

$$L = mvr = \frac{hr}{\lambda} \tag{1.5}$$

Putting (1.4) in (1.5) gives

$$L = mvr = \frac{nh}{2\pi} \tag{1.6}$$

(This is referred to as quantized angular momentum).

By using quantization of angular momentum, kinetic energy

$$\frac{n^2 h^2}{8\pi^2 mr^2} \tag{1.7}$$

(obtained by putting (1.6) in (1.2)).

Total energy of the classical orbit of hydrogen atom = potential energy + kinetic energy of the electron

Potential energy

$$U = -\frac{Ze^2}{4\pi \varepsilon_0 r}$$

Kinetic energy

$$T = \frac{Ze^2}{8\pi \varepsilon_0 r} \tag{1.8}$$

Total energy

$$T + U = -\frac{Ze^2}{8\pi \varepsilon_0 r} \tag{1.9}$$

Equating (1.2), (1.7), and (1.8) to the equation of kinetic energy

$$\text{Kinetic energy} = \frac{mv^2}{2} = \frac{(mvr)^2}{2mr^2} = \frac{n^2 h^2}{8\pi^2 mr^2} = \frac{Ze^2}{8\pi \varepsilon_0 r}$$

By substituting for $r = \frac{n^2 h^2 \varepsilon_0}{Z\pi m e^2} = \frac{n^2 a_0}{Z}$ in the equation of total energy in (1.9) gives

$$E = -\frac{Z^2 m e^4}{8 n^2 h^2 \varepsilon_0^2} = -\frac{13.6 Z^2}{n^2} \text{eV}$$

$$\ln r = \frac{n^2 h^2 \varepsilon_0}{Z\pi m e^2} = \frac{n^2 a_0}{Z};$$

$$a_0 = 0.539\text{Å} = \text{BohrRadius}$$

The Bohr's radius is defined as the *least distance from the nuclei at which a single electron revolves in an orbit which is at the lowest energy state.*

(OR)

The Bohr radius a_0 can be derived by equating.

The centrifugal force of an electron following a circular trajectory (in its orbit) around a proton and the electrostatic force experienced by the electron is given by

$$m\frac{v^2}{r} = \frac{q^2}{4\pi \varepsilon_o r^2}$$

where

m is the mass of the electron in kg,
v is the velocity of the electron in m/sec,
r is the radius of the orbit in m,
q is the charge (usually point charge when considered) in Coulomb, and
ε_o is the permittivity of free space $= 8.8541878176 \times 10^{-12}$ farads per meter (F/m).

According to DeBroglie's equation of wavelength,

$$\lambda = \frac{h}{p},$$

where lambda, λ is the wavelength in meters (m),

$$h = \text{Planck's constant} = 6.626 \times 10^{-34} \text{ JouleSec.} = 4.136 \times 10^{-15} \text{ eV.Sec}$$

$$p = \text{momentum} \frac{\text{kg.m}}{\text{Sec.}} = \text{mass} \times \text{velocity} = mv.$$

According to the standing wave condition, the circumference of an orbit of a particle (electron) is equal to the whole number times the associated wavelength.

$$2\pi r = n\lambda$$

For first orbit $2\pi r = \lambda$.

From $p = h/\lambda$ and $\lambda = 2\pi r$ one finds that

$$p = \frac{h}{2\pi r}$$

Therefore

$$\frac{mv^2}{r} = \frac{p^2}{rm} = \frac{\left(h/2\pi\right)^2}{mr^3} = \frac{q^2}{4\pi \varepsilon_o r^2}$$

On simplifying for the Bohr's radius r, we get

$$r = \frac{4\pi \varepsilon_o h^2}{mq^2},$$

this radius is represented by a_0. The numeric value is

$$a_0 = 0.539 \text{Å} = \text{BohrRadius}$$

The Bohr's radius is defined as the *least distance from the nuclei at which a single electron revolves in an orbit which is at the lowest energy state.*

Bohr's model assumes that the energy of the particles in an atom is restricted or confined to certain discrete values, i.e., the energy levels are *quantized.* This translates into the existence of only certain orbits with certain radii while intermediate orbits are not allowable and therefore do not exist. Fig. 1.1 illustrates Bohr's atomic model for the hydrogen atom [11].

In Bohr's hydrogen model, the number n is defined as the *quantum number* which takes the values of various positive integers; $n = 1, 2, 3 \ldots$ and each number corresponds to an *"energy state"* or *"energy level."* Fig. 1.2 illustrates the different energy levels [11].

The lowest energy level is referred to as ground state; the successive higher energy states are called first excited state, second excited state, and so on. Further, in the energy state (level) beyond the *"ionization potential"* the electron is no longer bound to the atom, forming a continuum. The *"ionization potential"* of a hydrogen atom is 13.6 eV (electron-volt).

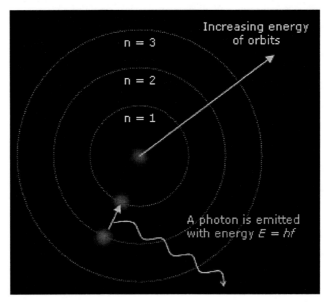

FIGURE 1.1: Bohr's atomic model

Atoms are excited or de-excited by absorbing or emitting the energy required to move between different orbits. Fig. 1.3 shows the excitation and de-excitation caused by photonic emissions [11].

One can comprehend from Bohr's model that an atom can absorb or emit only discrete energy "packets." This energy will follow the equation [12].

$$E = h\nu$$

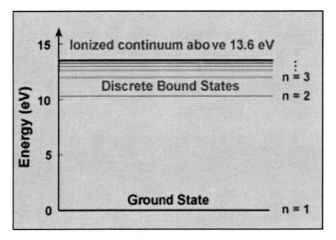

FIGURE 1.2: Quantized energy levels in hydrogen

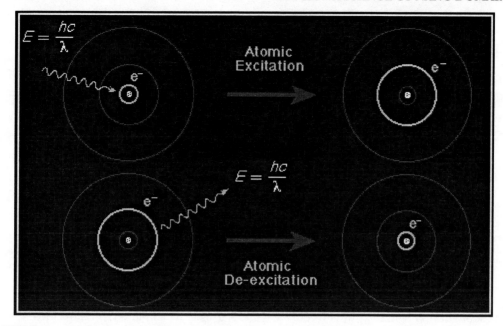

FIGURE 1.3: Excitation by absorption of light and de-excitation by emission of light

Also

$$E = \frac{hc}{\lambda} \quad \text{since} \quad v = \frac{c}{\lambda}$$

where,

E is the energy required for excitation or de-excitation,
h is Planck's constant,
v (pronounced nu) is the frequency (sec^{-1}),
c is the velocity of light (m sec^{-1}), and
λ is the wavelength (m).

1.5   COMPARISON OF PARTICLE BEHAVIOR AT NANO-SIZE TO MACRO SIZE: GOLD AND TITANIA

This section elucidates the importance and applications of NP of gold (AuNP) and titanium di-oxide (TiO_2–titania) nanoparticles—TNP. We start with a comparison of the macro size to the nano domain of each material to obtain an insight of the value of nanosize for various applications.

a) Gold Nanoparticles (AuNP)

Mining of gold and using it for various decorative and medical purposes has been of great interest since ancient times. With technological developments, the smelting of gold too took crucial turns thereby opening newer techniques of synthesis. In the present day gold nanoparticles (AuNP) seem to be of more interest than their macro counterparts, at least to the world of research. AuNP have interesting properties that scientists are able to exploit. Key properties of AuNP include their stability, non-toxicity, bio-compatibility, characteristic optical properties, and surface plasmon resonance (SPR) behavior. These provide the potential for unique catalytic and biological applications [13–15].

AuNP includes colloidal gold as well as thin film gold. The synthesis of colloidal gold is a highly reproducible robust process with capability of producing colloidal AuNP as small as 1.5 nm [15]. A popular application of colloidal gold is the use of 1.4 nm AuNP as an electronic switch to control the hybridization and re-hybridization of DNA by conjugating the AuNPs to the DNA [16].

Colloidal gold particles of different sizes emit visible light of different wavelengths. The smallest of gold NP will emit pink or purple while aggregated sample turns yellow [13]. Unlike metallic gold of micron size, AuNP has a unique property called the SPR. This SPR is being utilized as a popular tool in biological applications for enzyme kinetics (as in the Biacore instrument) or in combination with Raman spectroscopy.

SPR is excited at a metal or dielectric interface by a monochromatic light source. SPR is observed as a deep minimum in the p-polarized reflected light as the angle of incidence is increased. The plasmon, a ray of light bound onto a surface, propagates among the surface and presents itself as an electromagnetic field [17].

SPR can then be used to amplify refractive index changes due to the adsorptions of thin layers of materials (proteins, antigens, etc.) adsorbed on a film of metal. For instance a protein in a buffer, when adsorbed on the surface of a metallic gold film, produces a change in the refractive index of the film compared to the system with just the buffer. The difference between the refractive index of the buffer and that of the adsorbate is converted to mass of the adsorbate. The initial refractive index is characteristic of the metal used. AuNP or thin films of gold exhibit excellent SPR effects. This method is rapidly replacing tedious and time-consuming enzyme kinetics experiments to determine binding affinities of antigens and antibodies [17, 18].

The SP could be used as a probe in biological applications as it is very sensitive to environmental changes close to the interface. Popular biological and immunological sensing techniques have been developed with AuNP–SPR that is remote and non-destructive. Also SP finds excellent applications in surface enhanced spectroscopy for example in surface plasmon fluorescence spectroscopy and surface enhanced Raman spectroscopy (SERS) [18, 19].

b) Titanium Di-oxide Nanoparticles (TNP)—Titania (TiO$_2$)

TiO$_2$ (titania), the naturally occurring oxide of titanium, not available in pure form is often synthesized from the ilmenite or leuxocene ores. Of the various forms of titania, rutile, anatase, brookite, and titanium dioxide (B) are the most common. TNP have superior catalytic properties to micron size or larger titania particles. TNP being smaller have higher surface area to volume ratio and hence improved catalytic activity [20].

A number of techniques are used for the synthesis of nanoparticles of TiO$_2$, namely the sol-gel method, the microemulsion technique, and the flame oxidation method. The outstanding catalytic properties of TNP make it one of the dominant catalysts used in the decomposition of organic pollutants and also in water treatment plants [6, 21]. The photocatalytic applications of TNP including water cleansing and pollution disinfection are often triggered by exposure to visible or UV irradiation [6]. Doping of titania with metals and/or semiconductors further its photocatalytic activity, the identification and optimization of such parameters represent an active area of bionanotechnology's academic and industrial research as manifested by several recent publications [22–27].

1.6   ADVANTAGES OF SCALING DOWN—NANO-SIZE

The main advantages of scaling down to nano-size in biological application include the following and become very important in drug delivery applications [1, 28].

Nanoparticles are able to:

1. Accumulate in the tissue of mononuclear phagocyte system (MPS) (formerly RES).
2. Leave the vasculature through leaky angiogenic vessels and accumulate in tumor interstitia. (drug delivery + imaging).
3. Achieve enhanced permeability and retention effect (EPR effect).

As mentioned earlier the concept of targeted drug delivery goes hand in hand with nano-size only. Choosing a nano-model of application in targeted drug delivery involves various notable advantages including, stability of drug in targeted delivery, prevention of phagocytosis, easy/passive transport of drug vehicles across epithelia, high surface volume ratio and hence better performance & appropriate drug release at target sites [29–37]. Current trends in research focus on creating multifunctional NP for *in vivo* use, for non-invasive visualization of molecular markers for early stage disease, for targeted delivery of therapeutics, reduction of deleterious side effects, and interception and containment of lesions before they reach lethal stage, with minimal or no loss of quality of life [36–41].

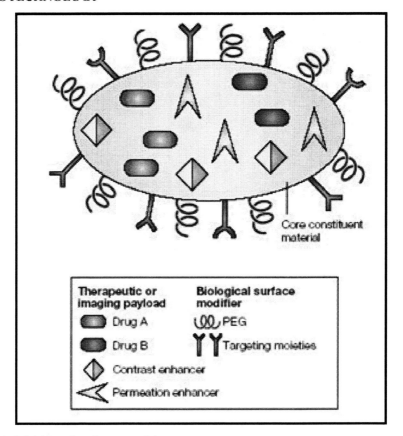

FIGURE 1.4: Multifunctional nanoparticle—nanovector

Fig. 1.4 is a schematic of a multifunctional nano-device (nanovector) comprising of two drugs, namely A and B for delivery, a contrast-enhancing agent for better imaging, a permeation enhancer for easier and sooner reachability to site, PEG coating to fool the immune system and targeting moieties for better specificity in targeting. All this being in the nanodomain will ensure quick passage of the vectors through the cells and pores and enable them to reach the disease target with ease [39].

Fig. 1.5 is a representation of the multifunctional targeting strategy in a tumor site. The nanovectors reach the tumor site by passing through the fenestrations of the angiogenic vasculature. One or more antibodies present in these nanovectors enable them to specifically and selectively bind to chosen sites. Having reached their specific sites, the nanovectors can be triggered to release their cytotoxic agents to create an antitumor action. The trigger could be accomplished by an external source (ultrasound, IR, MRI, etc.) or by using internal factors such as pH or temperature [39].

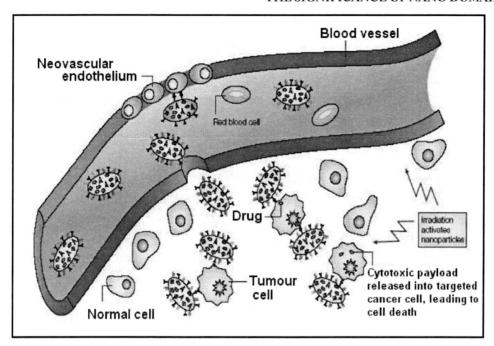

FIGURE 1.5: Multifunctional targeting strategy in a tumor site

REFERENCES

[1] H. Frieboes and J. Sinek, *Handbook of BioMEMS & Bio-Nanotechnology—Prospectus, Biological and Biomedical Nanotechnology: Nanotechnology in cancer drug therapy: a Biocomputational approach.* In *Onco-Imaging, Medicine-Hematology/Oncology.*, A. Lee, L. Lee, Eds. Berlin: Springer, vol. 1, pp. 435–460, 2006.

[2] P. Gerwins, E. Skoldenberg, L. Claesson-Welsh, "Function of fibroblast growth factors and vascular endothelial growth factors and their receptors in angiogenesis," *Crit. Rev. Oncol./Hematol.*, vol. **34** (3), p. 185, 2000.

[3] S. Muro, R. Wiewrodt, A. Thomas, L. Koniaris, S. M. Albelda, V. R. Muzykantov, M. Koval, A novel endocytic pathway induced by clustering endothelial ICAM-1 or PECAM-1. *J. Cell Sci.* vol. **116**(8), pp. 1599–1609, 2003.

[4] B. Peppas, L. Blanchette, O. James, Nanoparticle and targeted systems for cancer therapy. *Adv. Drug Deliv. Rev.* vol. **56**, pp. 1649–1659, 2004.

[5] A. Majumdar, Nanotechnology Research in Support of Homeland Security: Chemical, Biological, Radiological, and Explosive (CBRE) Detection and Protection. http://www.nano.gov/html/news/SpecialPapers/Nanotechnology%20Research%20in% 20support%20of%20Homeland%20Security_cbre.htm (10/09/2006),

[6] S. Ma, J. Zhou, Y. C. Kang, J. E. Reddic, D. A. Chen, Dimethyl methyl-phosphonate decomposition on Cu surfaces: supported Cu nanoclusters and films on TiO2 (110). *Langmuir* vol. **20**, pp. 9686–9694, 2004.

[7] G. Nagaveni, M. S. Sivalingam, Hegde; Giridharmadras, Photocatalytic degradation of organic compounds over combustion-synthesized nano-TiO2. *Environ. Sci. Technol.* vol. **38**, pp. 1600–1604, 2004.

[8] D. S. Goodsell, *Bionanotechnology: Lessons from Nature.* Wiley-Liss, (311), pp. 9–14, 2004.

[9] D. S. Goodsell, *Bionanotechnol. Lessons Nat.* (311), 103–116, 2004.

[10] V. P. Zharov, J.-W. Kim, D. T. Curiel, M. Everts, Self-assembling nanoclusters in living systems: application for integrated photothermal nanodiagnostics and nanotherapy. *Nanomedicine* vol. **1**(4), pp. 326–345, 2005.

[11] N. Bohr, Astronomy Lectures—The Bohr Model. http://csep10.phys.utk.edu/astr162/lect/light/bohr.html (10/10/2006),

[12] C. R. Nave, Hyperphysics: Planks Theory. http://hyperphysics.phy-astr.gsu.edu/hbase/whframe.html (10/10/2006),

[13] M.-C. Daniel, Didier, Gold nanoparticles: assembly, supra-molecular chemistry, quantum-size-related properties, and applications toward biology, catalysis, and nanotechnology. *Astruc Chem. Rev.* vol. **104**, pp. 293–346, 2004.

[14] I. El-Sayed, X. Huang, and M. El-Sayed, Surface plasmon resonance scattering and absorption of anti-EGFR antibody conjugated gold nanoparticles in cancer diagnostics: applications in oral cancer. *Nano Lett.* vol. **5**(5), pp. 829–834, 2005.

[15] K. V. Sarathy, G. Raina, R. T. Yadav, G. U. Kulkarni, C. N. R. Rao, Thiol-derivatized nanocrystalline arrays of gold, silver, and platinum. *J. Phys. Chem. B* vol. **101**, pp. 9876–9880, 1997.

[16] H. K. Schifferli, "DNA hybridization: electronic control," *Dekker Encyclopedia of Nanoscience and Nanotechnology.* Taylor & Francis Books, Oxford, UK, pp. 963–974, 2004.

[17] M. Zangeneh, R. Terrill, Surface plasmon spectra of silver and gold nanoparticle assemblies *Dekker Encyclopedia of Nanoscience and Nanotechnology*, Taylor & Francis Books, Oxford, UK, 2004.

[18] J. W. D. P. B. Attridge, J. K. Deacon, G. P. Davidson, Sensitivity enhancement of optical immunosensors by the use of a surface plasmon resonance fluoroimmunoassay. *Biosens. Bioelectron.* vol. **6**(3), pp. 201–214, 1991.

[19] Z. Salamon, Y. Wang, G. Tollin, H. A. MacLeod, Assembly and molecular organization of self-assembled lipid bilayers on solid substrates monitored by surface plasmon resonance spectroscopy. *Biochim. Biophys. Acta* vol. **1195**, pp. 267–275, 1994.

[20] S.-H. Lee, "Photocatalytic nanocomposites based on TiO2 and carbon nanotubes," *Doctoral Thesis*, University of Florida, Gainesville, 2004.

[21] C. N. Rusu, J. T. Yates Jr., Photooxidation of dimethyl methyl-phosphonate on TiO2 powder. *J. Phys. Chem. B* vol. **104**, pp. 12299–12305, 2000.

[22] A. Dawson, P. V. Kamat, Semiconductor-metal nanocomposites. photoinduced fusion and photocatalysis of gold-capped TiO_2 (TiO_2/Gold) nanoparticles. *J. Phys. Chem. B* vol. **105**(5), pp. 960–966, 2001.

[23] T. Hirakawa, P. V. Kamat, Charge separation and catalytic activity of $AgTiO^2$ core-shell composite clusters under UV-irradiation. *J. Am. Chem. Soc.* vol. **127**(11), pp. 3928–3934, 2005.

[24] K. S. Mayya, D. I. Gittins, F. Caruso, Gold-titania core-shell nanoparticles by polyelectrolyte complexation with a titania precursor. *Chem. Mater.* vol. **13**(11), pp. 3833–3836, 2001.

[25] V. Subramanian, E. Wolf, P. V. Kamat, Semiconductor-metal composite nanostructures. to what extent do metal nanoparticles improve the photocatalytic activity of TiO^2 films? *J. Phys. Chem. B* vol. **105**(46), pp. 11439–11446, 2001.

[26] V. Subramanian, E. E. Wolf, P. V. Kamat, Influence of metal/metal ion concentration on the photocatalytic activity of TiO^2 -Au composite nanoparticles *Langmuir* vol. **19**(2), pp. 469–474, 2003.

[27] V. Subramanian, E. E. Wolf, P. V. Kamat, Catalysis with TiO^2 /gold nanocomposites. effect of metal particle size on the Fermi level equilibration. *J. Am. Chem. Soc.* vol. **126** (15), pp. 4943–4950, 2004.

[28] M. Ferrari, "Cancer nanotechnology: opportunities and challenges," *Nat. Rev.-Cancer* vol. **5**, pp. 161–171, March 2005.

[29] L. Brannon-Peppas, J. O. Blanchette, Nanoparticle and targeted systems for cancer therapy. *Adv. Drug Deliv. Rev.* vol. **56**(11), pp. 1649–1659, 2004.

[30] P. Couvreur, et al., Nanotechnologies for drug delivery: Application to cancer and autoimmune diseases. *Prog. Solid State Chem.*, vol. **34**(2–4), pp. 231–235, 2006.

[31] R. Duncan, Nanomedicine gets clinical. *Mater. Today* vol. **8** (8, Supplement 1), p. 16, 2005.

[32] R. A. Freitas Jr., What is nanomedicine? *Nanomedicine* vol. **1** (1), pp. 2–9, 2005.

[33] A. Hughes Gareth, Nanostructure-mediated drug delivery. *Disease-a-month: DM* vol. **51**(6), pp. 342–61, 2005.

[34] E. S. Kawasaki, A. Player, Nanotechnology, nanomedicine, and the development of new, effective therapies for cancer. *Nanomedicine* vol. **1**(2), pp. 101–109, 2005.

[35] J. Kreuter, "Application of nanoparticles for the delivery of drugs to the brain," *Int. Congress Series* vol. **1277**, p. 85, 2005.

[36]   Y. Nishioka, H. Yoshino, Lymphatic targeting with nanoparticulate system. *Adv. Drug Deliv. Rev.* vol. **47**(1), p. 55, 2001.

[37]   J. E. Schnitzer, Vascular targeting as a strategy for cancer therapy. *N. Engl. J. Med.* vol. **339**(7), pp. 472–474, 1998.

[38]   S. Kim, Y. T. Lim, E. G. Soltesz, A. M. De Grand, J. Lee, A. Nakayama, J. A. Parker, T. Mihaljevic, R. G. Laurence, D. M. Dor, L. H. Cohn, M. G. Bawendi, J. V. Frangioni, Near-infrared fluorescent type II quantum dots for sentinel lymph node mapping. *Nat. Biotech.* vol. **22**(1), p. 93, 2004.

[39]   M. Ferrari, "Cancer nanotechnology: opportunities and challenges," *Nat. Rev.—Cancer* vol. **5**, pp. 161–171, 2005.

[40]   A. Wickline Samuel, M. Lanza Gregory, Nanotechnology for molecular imaging and targeted therapy. *Circulation* vol. **107**(8), pp. 1092–5, 2003.

[41]   W. Zhao, Ehrlich's magic nanobullets. *Nanomedicine* vol. **1**(3), p. 238, 2005.

CHAPTER 2

Nano Drug Delivery

IMPORTANCE OF NANOSIZE IN DRUG DELIVERY

This chapter elucidates the fundamentals of drug delivery systems, starting with traditional drug delivery vehicles and routes of delivery. The need for nano-vehicles and the advantages they offer is explained with specific examples. The concept of targeted delivery and the role of nano technology in combination with targeted delivery are also covered.

2.1 CONVENTIONAL DRUG DELIVERY

2.1.1 First Pass Effect

Despite the discovery of a large number of active compounds as potential drugs, very few of these research products achieve clinical success mostly due to problems related to their bioavailability. Bioavailability [1] depends on the route of administration of a particular drug and depends on the rate of absorption and metabolism of the drug by the body [2].

The most popular route adapted for the intake of a drug is the peroral route better known as the oral route. The drug stays in the stomach for a considerable time during the process of digestion. Various body fluids such as gastric acids interact with the pill in the stomach. After digestion, the pill, along with other food particles that are broken down in the stomach, goes through the intestine where it is absorbed through the intestinal walls into the enterohepatic circulation where the pill, now broken down to its constituent drugs, is taken to the liver for detoxification. The process of the drug's encounter with the liver is referred to as the *first pass effect* [3]. After having undergone the first pass effect the drug completely mixes with the blood stream. Fig. 2.1 [3] depicts, step by step, various barriers encountered by an orally delivered drug [2]. The first pass effect is of great significance to the pharmaceutical and health care industries because it greatly determines the fate of a drug. A schematic of classical drug delivery is shown in Fig. 2.2 where the drug is seen to be depleted from the body through metabolism and excretion [3].

Oral administration in strict terms refers to the process where the drug is directly absorbed into the circulation through the mouth itself, by placing the pill under the tongue, or placing it between the gingiva and the cheeks [4]. This mode is also known as the buccal route. The

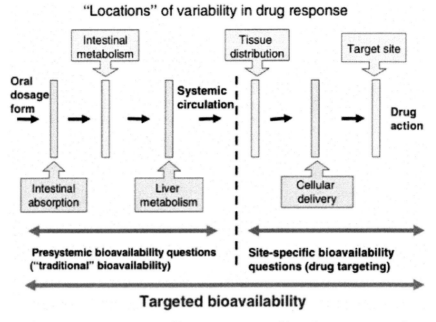

FIGURE 2.1: Schematic representation of barriers encountered by a drug en route to the target site

mouth is then an active participant in drug absorption; the drug easily diffuses into the mucous membrane and reaches the circulatory system via the jugular vein. Although, in the buccal route of drug delivery, there is a chance of partial drug swallowing, this route has the considerable advantage of bypassing the first pass effect and escaping the strong acidic environment in the stomach. Overcoming the first pass effect or bypassing it has become a popular trend in many drug delivery applications, widely practiced today.

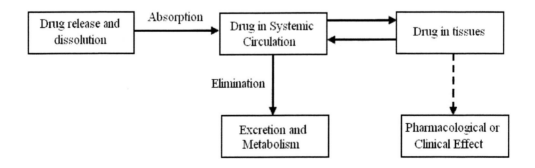

FIGURE 2.2: Schematic representation of drug and its pharmacological effect

TABLE 2.1: Various routes of drug delivery and forms of drug administered

ROUTE OF DRUG DELIVERY	STATE/FORM OF DRUG DELIVERED
Oral	Pill, capsule, liquid, suspension, cream
Nasal	Liquid, aerosol, vapor
Ophthalmic	Liquid, gel, cream, ointment, suspension
Parenteral {all non-Gastro-intestinal routes qualify}	Liquid (by injection—including intravenal)
Topical and transdermal	Ointment, gel, foam, cream, powder, liquid
Pulmonary (through lungs)	Deep nasal inhalations of liquid, aerosol
Vaginal	Suppositories, cream, foam, solutions, gel, ointment
Rectal	Suppositories (mostly torpedo shaped), cream, foam, solution, gel, ointment

2.1.2   Routes of Delivery

The choice of appropriate route of delivery is often based on the type and location of the injury or disease. Table 2.1 gives a brief idea of the various routes and forms of drug delivery. It is notable that all the following routes of delivery, except oral, bypass the first pass effect [3, 5–12].

The ultimate consideration for a drug's efficacy is its availability at the target site, referred to as "bioavailability" [2]. In the case of oral administration there are two distinct levels of bioavailability, a systemic response and a site-specific cellular availability response. Both are critical not only because they determine the functionality of a drug but also because they control the side effects of a particular formulation.

Fig. 2.3 [2] illustrates various physiological factors that interfere with a drug; this includes protein binding, receptor affinity, membrane permeability, protein expression, gene regulation, and others, which depend on the physicochemical properties and the site of the drug action [2].

Factors such as drug transport and drug metabolism are determined by their dosage and the physiological conditions. In a collective manner, all the above-mentioned factors result in determining the bioavailability of the drug which initiates a pharmacological response in the target site. In case of over dosage, toxicological and inflammatory responses are provoked at the target site.

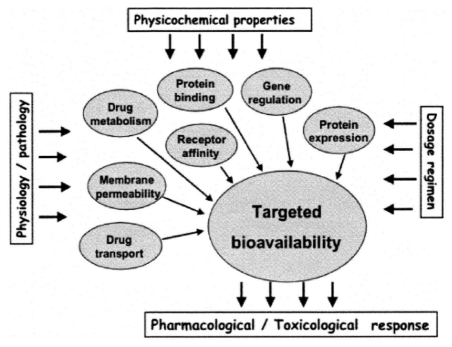

FIGURE 2.3: Schematic representation of factors that influence the bioavailability of a drug

2.2   TARGETED DRUG DELIVERY

One approach to improve bioavailability is targeted drug delivery, avoiding over dosage-toxicity [13] and consequential inflammatory response [14, 15]. Targeted delivery aims to achieve perfection by delivering the right amount at only the site of disease or injury. One of the prime aspects of a competent targeted-drug delivery system is the selection of an appropriate delivery profile [2]. The delivery profile is usually a plot of the concentration of drug delivered from the vehicle with respect to time. The drug delivery profile is characteristic of the type of drug, the type of drug vehicle, and the physiological factors at the delivery site. For instance, pore size, thickness, geometry, drug loading, temperature, surface roughness, bio-degradation, etc. of the drug vehicle determine the amount of drug that is released, thus controlling the profile of delivery. Drugs can be classified into organics, carbohydrates, surfactants, polymers, lipids, fats, amino acids, peptides, and proteins [16]. This choice of a drug determines how it will interact with its delivery vehicle and hence the delivery profile, for instance hydrophobicity or hydrophilicity plays a crucial role in releasing of the drug.

Table 2.2 [16] lists a few notable drug delivery vehicles of interest to bionanotechnology and their corresponding sizes. Others include metal nanoshells [17], dendrimers [18], nanofibers, nanotubes etc.

TABLE 2.2: Microparticulate colloidal carrier systems

NANOSIZE DRUG SIZE OF DELIVERY	DELIVERY VEHICLES VEHICLE (NM)
Nanocapsules	50–200
Uni-lamellar liposomal vesicles	25–200
Nanoparticles	25–200
Microemulsions	20–50

2.3 CHEMISTRY OF DRUG DELIVERY VEHICLES

2.3.1 Nanocapsules

Nanocapsules are polymeric membranes with an oily or aqueous core. They can be defined as a vesicular system in which "drug is confined to an aqueous or oily cavity surrounded by a single polymeric membrane" [19]. They are colloidal carriers applied for drug delivery [20]. Usually the nanocapsules contain an outer surfactant adsorption layer as shown in Fig. 2.4. Polyalkylcyanoacrylates and poly-lactides are some of the polymers used for the outer coating. While the core of the vehicle comprises of "soya bean oil or other triglycerides having long and medium chain fatty acids" [20]. Nanocapsule of polyisobutylcyanoacrylate (PIBCA) finds extensive applications in drug delivery.

2.3.2 Unilamellar Liposomal Vesicles

Liposomes are one of the popular delivery vehicles that are used in the modern day. Extensive application of liposomal delivery for tumor and cancer therapy has caused much development

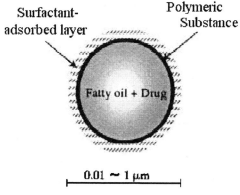

FIGURE 2.4: Construction of a nanocapsule

and widespread know-how of factors that facilitate efficient delivery in liposomal vehicles [21]. They are *"vesicular colloidal particles composed of self-assembled amphiphillic molecules"* [21]. They have both hydrophilic as well as hydrophobic groups in them, thus enabling a possible self-assembly in an aqueous medium [21]. Liposomes consist of "neutral or anionic lipids" which may be synthetic or natural, e.g., natural lipids include lecithins, sphingomyelins etc., which are extracted from egg yolk, soya beans etc, while their synthetic counterparts include chains of dimyristoyl, dipalmitoyl, distearoyl, and dioleoyl. Functionally liposomes can be classified as conventional, cationic, stealth, and targeted liposomes [21].

Size is a prominent factor that determines the targeting efficiency and the associated therapeutic effects in liposomes. It has been substantiated that the very size determines the liposomal accumulation in tumor site, efficacy of therapy, level of toxicity, cross vessel permeation, and overall transport in the body [14]. Further, it has been revealed that lesser the size better the extent of targeting and efficacy of therapy which can be associated with the amount of drug reaching the tumor site in particular. Liposomes of 100 nm size and less have exhibited better targeting and accumulation in tumor site [14].

2.3.3 Nanoparticles

Nanoparticles (NP) are collection of several atoms of a particular element in a given fashion. Usually the NP is in the submicron range, mostly less than 200 nm which are of high interest to bionanotech [19]. NP of gold, silver, zinc oxide, titania etc. finds excellent applications in bionanotech. When functionalized with antibodies, these nanoparticles can perform targeted delivery [22]. Usually NP is employed as drug delivery vehicles and biomarkers of tumors and cancer cells. Having high "enhanced permeability and retention" (EPR), they are much preferred for tumor and cancer therapy [19]. Alginate NPs are one other type of the class of nanoparticles being extensively used for drug delivery [23]. They are made of tiny calcium/sodium alginate gel. Notable of the bio-imaging nanoparticles include polystyrene fluorescent NP. Muller book [23].

2.3.4 Microemulsions

The microemulsions are "clear, stable, isotropic mixtures of oil, water and surfactant, frequently in combination with a cosurfactant" [24]. Microemulsion when loaded with drug serves as efficient drug delivery vehicles. Spherical micelle, rod-shaped micelle, hexagonal phase, lamellar phase, reverse hexagonal phase, and reverse micelle are the most commonly observed "self-association" structures of micelle. Fig. 2.5 shows the commonly seen microstructures in the microemulsions [24].

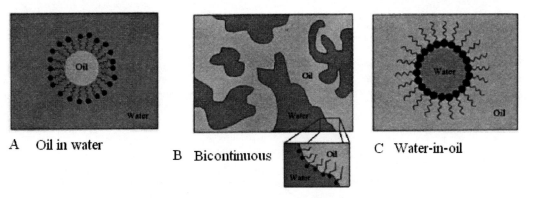

FIGURE 2.5: Various microstructures in a microemulsion

2.4   DELIVERY PROFILES

The delivery profile of a drug delivery system determines the bioavailability of a drug at a given time [2]. A classical drug delivery profile is shown in Fig. 2.6, where two important types of delivery, one shot delivery (single dose) and multiple dose delivery, are depicted [2]. A single dosage drug, when delivered, attains a concentration peak in its release profile and then decays.

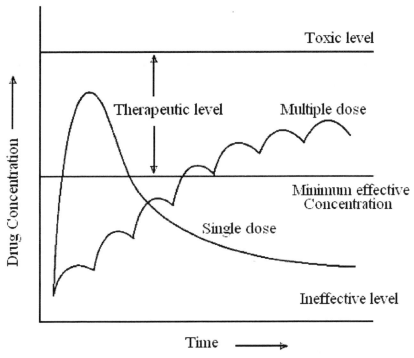

FIGURE 2.6: Plot of drug concentration versus time for single and multiple doses

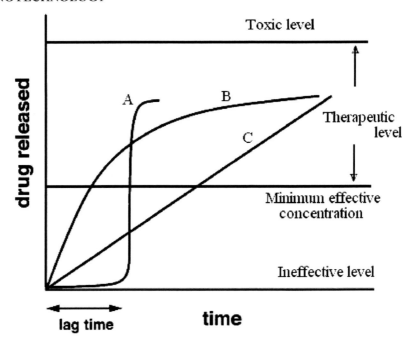

FIGURE 2.7: Various controlled release profiles. (A) Initial time lag release profile, (B) sustained release profile, and (C) linear time release profile

A multiple dose delivery has several peaks in its concentration/release profile and then falls down as time goes on. In both single and multiple doses, it is important to distinguish the different levels of bioavailability shown in Fig. 2.6; insufficient level, therapeutic level, and toxic level. An ideal delivery profile should achieve constant delivery in the therapeutic region, with a safe margin below the toxic level and above the ineffective level [2].

The delivery profiles shown in Fig. 2.6 are not the preferred. Different types of controlled delivery profiles are depicted in Fig. 2.7 [3].

The most appropriate selection for a drug delivery would be that of the sustained release because it lies mainly in the therapeutic region. Fig. 2.7(A) is a type of controlled release where the initial drug release is nearly zero and then there is a sharp rise in release whereas in Fig. 2.7(B) a sustained release is observed while Fig. 2.7(C) shows a linear time release profile. Fig. 2.8 shows release profiles of a prolonged release and controlled releases which have a major drug release within in the *Therapeutic Level* [2]. Often in controlled drug release, the main factor of interest is drug release in the therapeutic region.

The controlled release drug delivery systems can be subdivided into the following four categories:

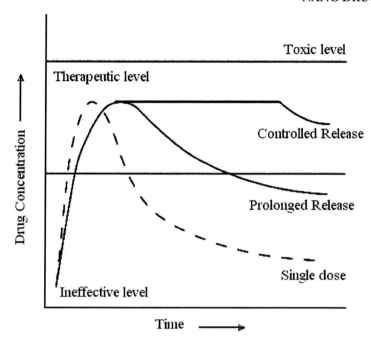

FIGURE 2.8: Plot of drug concentration versus time for different release systems

2.4.1   Rate-Preprogrammed Drug Delivery Systems

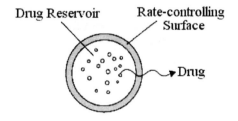

2.4.2   Activation-Modulated Drug Delivery Systems

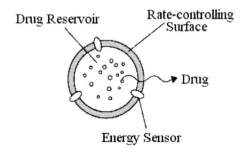

2.4.3   Feedback-Regulated Drug Delivery Systems

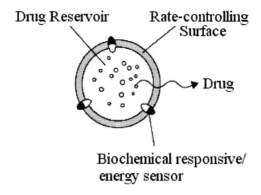

2.4.4   Site-Targeting Drug Delivery Systems

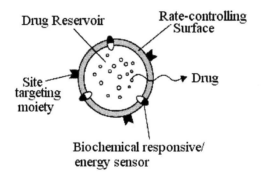

2.5   THE ROLE OF NANOTECHNOLOGY IN DRUG DELIVERY

An ideal drug delivery vehicle would be capable to navigate on its own, hunt, and find every single diseased cell and destroy it. In chronic diseases, an implanted miniature drug reservoir would administer life-saving drugs in the right amount at the right time. We would like to see that the drug was able to kill the diseased cells without harmful radiation and we would like to help control the navigation of delivery vehicles with precision [25] at will without invasive procedures.

The above wish list is neither imaginary nor utopian; it is very close to reality in a few years with the advances and research focus in bionanotechnology. The breakthroughs of bio-nanotechnology in the area of drug delivery [25, 26] have been some of the most remarkable applications of nanotechnology in medicine and include immuno-isolated nano porous implants with embedded pancreatic cells delivering insulin for diabetic patients, polarity-based gated nanosieves for selected ion transport, externally controlled nanoshell delivery vehicles for precision targeting, single virus detectors, gene engineered biological robots, artificial RBC [27].

2.5.1   Transdermal

Experimental researches over years have been exploring the possibility and extent of realization of transdermal drug delivery. The first successful model of transdermal delivery was a scopolamine patch created in 1979. There have been earlier studies on the barriers to a transdermal delivery dating back to as early as 1924. In the United States, annual expenditure in drug delivery in more than $3 billions, such a high profile industry namely health care is not driven for mere disease and injury therapies but also for novel applications such an nicotine delivery [28]. The consequences of delivery nicotine by patches through skin have led to creation of more than one million smokers who were otherwise [28].

The major challenges faced in the transdermal application are the possibility of an efficient and easy delivery of drug through skin's major barrier such as stratum corneum (SC), the epidermis etc. Of the two mentioned, SC is the major challenge. The stratum corneum is 10–15 µm thick, while epidermis is 50–100 µm thick and the dermis layer is about 2–3 mm thick. Usually, a drug/vehicle for a transdermal delivery cannot easily pass through the SC. [29].

Nanotechnology plays a promising role in transdermal applications. The smaller size enables easy permeation. Further, surface modifications enable targeted delivery. The present day research explores the use of certain external agencies in combination with nano vehicles for delivery. Notable among them are chemical enhancement, electricity assisted electroporation, low frequency ultrasound, PW mediated, and micro needles [28].

In order to deliver drugs at therapeutic useful rates, micro needles which are in the size of a micron dimensions were designed [30]. capable of delivering drugs when poked into the skin. Drugs made of nanoparticles can efficiently be delivered directly into the epidermis via this method. Needles of different sizes, shapes, and materials namely stainless steel, titanium, and silicon wafers are available. These needles usually have a small radius tip with thick walls. [30] which have lesser probability of fracture when using. To further improve this, micro needle arrays were designed which would have about 480 needles of each 430 µm long within a 2 sq. cm. area. Although this method could not be considered in case of skin burns and injuries, it is promising otherwise [30].

The application of PW facilitates temporary poration in the SC and allows the drugs/vehicles to easily pass through. Moreover it is painless, efficient, and has immediate recovery with regard to SC functionality by resuming to its normal character of being a high barrier [29]. The duration of exposure to PW is a crucial factor as it is directly proportional to the permeation through SC. The successful establishment of delivering 100 nm latex beads shows promising future for the delivery of DNA plasmids and proteins into the epidermis. Pressure waves (PW) generated from intense laser radiation applied on skin for transdermal drug delivery are gaining interest. It has been substantiated to show better permeation of drug vehicles across the stratum corneum (SC) and cell membrane, and ease of the very process of delivery [29]. A typical PW for the transdermal delivery would be of several hundred bars, a PW of 300–1000 bar for a period of 100 ns to 1 µm; here insulin was delivered to control blood glucose level [29]. The damages that might be caused due to PW are minimal and can be reduced by appropriate design of PWs [29].

Instead of having a traditional approach, even targeting the sweat glands and hair follicle being explored which show a sooner and better delivery when compared to overall skin flux [31], they work as shunt routes.

Other transdermal applications include dendrimers which are extensively used to deliver drugs, vaccines, and chemotherapeutic agents for cancer therapy [18]. Some of the dendrimer-based bionano applications include gene delivery, targeted cancer therapy, *in vivo* diagnoses (MRI), antiinfective agent delivery, vaccine and peptide delivery and drug delivery through oral and transdermal routes and ocular applications [18].

2.5.2   Blood Brain Barrier

BBB is one of the chief barriers usually not easy for to break in for drugs such as anticancer agents, antibiotics, peptides, oligo-molecules, and macromolecules [32]. The inaccessibility of drug to the brain tissues is attributed to the presence of "tight junctions between the endothelial cell linings in the brain blood vessels" [32]. Further, any drug across the endothelial lining is transported back into the blood stream by means of ABC transporters which are referred to as the "very active drug transport system." Thus, cranial drug delivery seems to be a major challenge in the medical world.

The transcytotic vesicular mechanism enables the transport of large molecules, while "specific transport systems for solute uptake are present on apical and basal membranes" but the efflux transporters of broader specificity are also present [33]. Efflux transporters do so with lipid-soluble drugs making them unreachable from the CNS. The dynamic of brain interstitial fluid (ISF) and the disease-caused BBB dysfunction contribute to the complication [33] of choosing a therapy. After all considerations, the drug vehicle interacts with the above-mentioned barriers at various point of time.

Nanoparticles provide to be an attractive solution to the BBB issue. Nanoparticles of smaller size when functionalized or suitably surface modified, mimicking LDL, bind to their specific receptors and diffuse into the endothelial cells ultimately reaching the interior of brain [34]. Hence the size and surface modification/functionalization enable the transport of nanodelivery vehicles across the BBB. However, the possibility of unintended intrusion via BBB into the brain is widely speculated; thus there must be high selectivity with regard to any uptake via BBB to avoid the unwelcome particles.

One of the successful establishments of drug delivery to brain includes the delivery of nanoparticles coated by polysorbate 80. Nanoparticles of drug vehicles coated with polysorbate 80 showed better uptake across BBB [32]. A notable instance was, during delivery of doxorubicin where the drug level in brain was in the ratio of 60:1 for the polysorbate-coated delivery versus the non-coated respectively [32].

With regard to nano drug delivery the possibility of delivery vehicles crossing the BBB can be reasoned to [33], an increased retention of the nanoparticles in the brain capillaries along with adsorption to the capillary walls could cause high concentration gradient facilitating the transport across the endothelial cells and ultimate delivery to the brain, "a general surfactant effect characterized by a solubilization of the endothelial cell membrane lipids that would lead to membrane fluidization and an enhanced drug permeability through the blood–brain barrier" [33], nanoparticles reaching the openings in tight junctions between endothelial cells could permeate either in free form or in bound form together with the nanoparticles, endocytosed NP releasing drug within the cells and delivered into brain, nano vehicles could be transcytosed through endothelial cells into brain, polysorbate 80 coating on nano vehicles could inhibit the efflux system. As mentioned earlier the NP delivery vehicle confronts the above-mentioned mechanism individually or collectively, hence the reason for a nano vehicle entering the brain could be attributed to one of these mechanisms or a combination of them.

2.6   ADVANTAGES OF TARGETED DRUG DELIVERY SYSTEMS

Targeted drug delivery systems are the future in drug delivery due to their specificity and efficacy. The benefit that one reaps through opting for a targeted drug delivery system includes protected payload and improved therapeutic index which is a comparison of the amount of drug that causes the therapeutic effect to the amount that causes toxic effects. Quantitatively, it is the ratio of the dose required to produce the toxic effect and the therapeutic dose. Also, targeted delivery enables increased specific localization, decreased toxic side effects, reduced dose, modulated pharmacokinetics, controlled bio-distribution, and importantly improved patient compliance.

REFERENCES

[1]   A. Kidane, P. P. Bhatt, "Recent advances in small molecule drug delivery," *Curr. Opin. Chem. Biol.*, vol. **9**(4), pp. 347–351, 2005.

[2]   T. S. BingheWang, Richard Soltero., *Drug Delivery: Principles and Applications (Textbook)* Wiley-Interscience, NJ. 2005, pp. 57–83 (462).

[3] L. S. A. B. C. Yu, Dekker Pharmaceutical Technology: Biopharmaceutics. Dekker Encyclopedias, Taylor and Francis Books, NY–USA. 2002.

[4] J. C. McElnay, C. M. Hughes, *Encyclopedia of Pharmaceutical Technology: Drug Delivery—Buccal Route*. Dekker Encyclopedias, Taylor and Francis Books, NY–USA. (April 28).

[5] M. J. Akers, *Encyclopedia of Pharmaceutical Technology: Drug Delivery—Parenteral Route*. Dekker Encyclopedias—Taylor and Francis Books, NY–USA. (May 8).

[6] M. C. A. L. W. H. Bhagat, *Encyclopedia of Pharmaceutical Technology: Drug Delivery—Ophthalmic Route*. Dekker Encyclopedias—Taylor and Francis Books, NY–USA. (May 8).

[7] R. Bommer, *Encyclopedia of Pharmaceutical Technology: Drug Delivery Nasal Route*. Dekker Encyclopedias—Taylor and Francis Books, NY–USA. (May 8).

[8] J. H. R. J. A. Fix, *Encyclopedia of Pharmaceutical Technology: Drug Delivery—Rectal Route*. Dekker Encyclopedias—Taylor and Francis Books, NY–USA. (May 8).

[9] B. N. S. K. H. Kim, *Encyclopedia of Pharmaceutical Technology: Drug Delivery—Oral Route*. Dekker Encyclopedias—Taylor and Francis Books, NY–USA. (May 8).

[10] Y. W. C. C. H. Lee, *Encyclopedia of Pharmaceutical Technology: Drug Delivery—Vaginal Route*. Dekker Encyclopedias—Taylor and Francis Books, NY–USA. (May 8).

[11] M. T. Newhouse, *Encyclopedia of Pharmaceutical Technology: Drug Delivery—Pulmonary Route*. Dekker Encyclopedias—Taylor and Francis Books, NY–USA. (May 8).

[12] K. A. Walters, *Encyclopedia of Pharmaceutical Technology: Drug Delivery—Topical and Transdermal Route*. Dekker Encyclopedias—Taylor and Francis Books, NY–USA (May 8).

[13] F. Chellat, Y. Merhi, A. Moreau, L. H. Yahia, Therapeutic potential of nanoparticulate systems for macrophage targeting, *Biomaterials*, vol. **26**(35), pp. 7260–7275, 2005.

[14] A. Nagayasu, K. Uchiyama, H. Kiwada, The size of liposomes: a factor which affects their targeting efficiency to tumors and therapeutic activity of liposomal antitumor drugs, *Adv. Drug Deliv. Rev.*, vol. **40**, (1–2), p. 75, 1999.

[15] A. Wickline Samuel, M. Lanza Gregory, Nanotechnology for molecular imaging and targeted therapy, *Circulation*, vol. **107**(8), pp. 1092–5, 2003.

[16] D. R. Karsa, R. A. Stephenson, *Chemical Aspects of Drug Delivery System*. Bradford: The Royal Society of Chemistry, pp. 1–10, 1996.

[17] O. Bomati-Miguel, M. P. Morales, P. Tartaj, J. Ruiz-Cabello, P. Bonville, M. Santos, X. Zhao, S. Veintemillas-Verdaguer, Fe-based nanoparticulate metallic alloys as contrast agents for magnetic resonance imaging, *Biomaterials* vol. **26**(28), pp. 5695–5703, 2005.

[18] R. Duncan, L. Izzo, Dendrimer biocompatibility and toxicity. *Adv. Drug Deliv. Rev.*, vol. **57**(15), p. 2215, 2005.

[19] I. Brigger, C. Dubernet, P. Couvreur, Nanoparticles in cancer therapy and diagnosis, *Adv. Drug Deliv. Rev.*, vol. **54**(5), pp. 631–651, 2002.

[20] Y. Nishioka, H. Yoshino, Lymphatic targeting with nanoparticulate system, *Adv. Drug Deliv. Rev.*, vol. **47**(1), p. 55, 2001.

[21] D. D. Lasic, *Liposomes in Gene Delivery*. Boca Raton, FL: CRC Press, 1997, pp. 67–113.

[22] P. Couvreur, et al., Nanotechnologies for drug delivery: Application to cancer and autoimmune diseases, *Prog. Solid State Chem.* vol. **34**(2–4), pp. 231–235, 2006.

[23] J. E. Diederichs, R. H. Muller, *Future Strategies for Drug Delivery with Particulate Systems*. Stuttgart-Germany: Medpharm GmbH Scientific Publishers, pp. 29–45, 1998.

[24] M. J. Lawrence, G. D. Rees, Microemulsion-based media as novel drug delivery systems, *Adv. Drug Deliv. Rev.*, vol. **45**(1), p. 89, 2000.

[25] E. S. Kawasaki, A. Player, Nanotechnology, nanomedicine, and the development of new, effective therapies for cancer, *Nanomedicine*, vol. **1**(2), pp. 101–109, 2005.

[26] R. Duncan, Nanomedicine gets clinical, *Mater. Today*, vol. **8**(8, Supplement 1), p. 16, 2005.

[27] R. A. Freitas, Jr., What is nanomedicine? *Nanomedicine*, vol. **1**, (1) pp. 2–9, 2005.

[28] R. Langer, Transdermal drug delivery: past progress, current status, and future prospects, *Adv. Drug Deliv. Rev.*, vol. **56**(5), p. 557, 2004.

[29] A. G. Doukas, N. Kollias, Transdermal drug delivery with a pressure wave, *Adv. Drug Deliv. Rev.*, vol. **56**(5), p. 559, 2004.

[30] M. R. Prausnitz, Microneedles for transdermal drug delivery. *Adv. Drug Deliv. Rev.*, vol. **56**(5), p. 581, 2004.

[31] B. W. Barry, Drug delivery routes in skin: a novel approach, *Adv. Drug Deliv. Rev.*, vol. **54** (Supplement 1), p. S31, 2002.

[32] J. Kreuter, Application of nanoparticles for the delivery of drugs to the brain, *Int. Congress Series*, vol. **1277**, p. 85, 2005.

[33] N. J. Abbott, Physiology of the blood-brain barrier and its consequences for drug transport to the brain, *Int. Congress Series*, vol. **1277**, p. 3, 2005.

[34] P. H. M. Hoet, I. Brueske-Hohlfeld, O. V. Salata, Nanoparticles-known and unknown health risks, *J. Nanobiotechnol.*, vol. **2**(1), pp. 12–17, 2004.

CHAPTER 3

BioNanoimaging

QUANTUM DOTS, ULTRASOUND CONTRAST AGENTS, AND MAGNETIC NANOPARTICLES

Background: The use of nanoparticles as biomarkers covers a broad range of materials and applications. Of the today's most popular contemporary bionano imaging applications, quantum dots (QDs), the ultrasound contrast agents (UCA), and the magnetic nanoparticles are the chief. Quantum dots are based on fluorescence optical properties, ultrasound contrast agents on differential absorption of ultrasound energy, and magnetic nanoparticles on unique super-paramagnetic properties associated with their small size. Applications can be in diagnostic imaging or targeted delivery or in novel multifunctional approaches. This chapter covers the basic function and properties of these materials and highlights their key applications.

3.1 QUANTUM DOTS

Quantum dots are nearly spherical, luminescent nanosized crystals made of semiconductor materials [1], of the order of 2–10 nm comprising 200–10 000 atoms [2]. Their optical properties are size-dependent [1]. A decrease in the crystal size causes an increase in energy shift between the absorbing and the emitting state [1]. Optical excitation across the band gap in a semiconductor depends on the size of the crystal even for larger crystals, as large as those comprising 10 000 atoms. A similar trend can be expected with the quantum dots which are often far too small with a minimum of 200 atoms extending to a maximum of 10 000 atoms [1, 2]. The band gaps of such nanocrystals are often tunable to the interest of the user, for instance a CdS crystal can be tuned between 2.5 and 4 eV [1].

Optical tunability [3, 4], better photostability, [3] and multicolor [5] light emission position QDs as the preferred fluorescent probes for dynamic live cell imaging tool and *in vivo* animal models [6–8]. They have unparalleled sensitivity and spatial resolution [2], compared to the organic fluorophores currently available. QDs with organic capping perform even better; these QDs usually have a core crystal with an inorganic capping with outer organic group which help during QD conjugation for functionalization [1]. For instance, a ZnS capped [7, 9] CdS

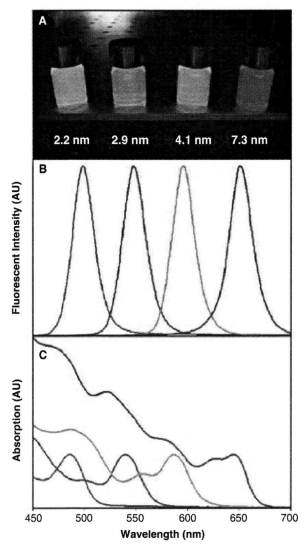

FIGURE 3.1: (A) Fluorescent images of CdS QDs using a 365 nm source. Sizes are 2.2 nm (blue), 2.9 nm (green), 4.1 nm (orange), and 7.3 nm (red) respectively. (B) Fluorescent spectra of the QDs indicating narrow emission spectra with minimal overlap; excitation of 400 nm. (C) The broad absorption spectra of these same four CdS QD's suggests the possibility of using a wide spectrum source for excitation (both absorption and emission spectra are plotted in AU—arbitrary units)

QD is 20 times brighter than rhodamine (a popular organic dye) and at the same time 100 times more stable to photobleaching [10].

Fig. 3.1 depicts CdS quantum dots of different sizes and how each size corresponds to a different color [2]. The same figure demonstrates the emission and absorption spectra of CdS

QDs in the presence of a UV source [2]. Further Fig. 3.1 indicates that the QDs have narrow wavelength and could be used with an exciting source having a wide spectrum.

QDs synthesis was first pioneered by Efros and Ekimov in the early 1980s [11–13]. Usually QD synthesis is followed by subsequent processes that functionalize the nanoparticles to become bio-active. The first step is the synthesis of the semiconductor core where a semiconductor precursor is chosen to synthesize a core. The chosen semiconductor determines the wavelength of the QD as being characteristic of the material chosen. Around the core, a shell is grown or capped such that the shell material processes a wider band gap than the core, thus providing higher electronic insulation, enhanced photoluminescence efficiency, and higher immunity to oxidation and degradation. This phase is referred to as *shell growth phase* [2].

The third phase of the QD synthesis is the *aqueous stabilization*. Attaining aqueous solubility is a prerequisite to enable use of the QDs for biological applications. Two different approaches are undertaken: either the QDs are synthesized in an aqueous solution or they are synthesized in an organic phase later followed by a phase transfer [2]. The latter method is often preferred due to its superior monodispersity, crystallinity, and high fluorescent efficiency. Finally, the QDs are conjugated with biological agents such as proteins, peptides, small organic molecules, and nucleic acids, thereby rendering them bioactive; this step is referred to as bio-conjugation [2].

Bioconjugation dictates the role and targeting of QDs in cellular and tissue applications by determining its affinity to a particular subcellular location or other biological entity. Usually, after aqueous stabilization, most QDs are covered with carboxylic groups. The carboxylic group plays a crucial role during bioconjugation reactions by forming a covalent bond with the amine groups of biomolecules participating in the bioconjugation. Most QDs are negatively charged and are dispersed in basic or neutral buffers. Hence, a positive biomolecule could be coated on the QDs based on the electrostatic interaction. Fig. 3.2 schematically describes various methods of bioconjugation [2]. The four methods depicted in Fig. 3.2 are coupling to QD surface, covalent coupling electrostatic attraction, and receptor-ligand binding where every method aims at coupling of biomolecules to the QD surface. The QDs shown in Fig. 3.2 are made water soluble by adding mercaptoacetic acid.

QDs can be used for the study of live cell single-molecule [14] dynamics, monitoring of intracellular protein–protein interactions, disease detection in deeper tissues, detection of cancer/tumor cells based on selective binding of bioconjugated QDs to known cancer biomarkers, and much more [2].

Fig. 3.3 shows green QDs conjugated to streptavidin, emitting green fluorescence. The image shows F-actins of fixed fibroblasts. Fig. 3.4 shows the image of cellular uptake of QD-cationic peptide conjugates [2]. The red-fluorescent (CdSe)ZnS QDs were incubated with a monolayer of living human cancer cells. The QDs were previously conjugated with

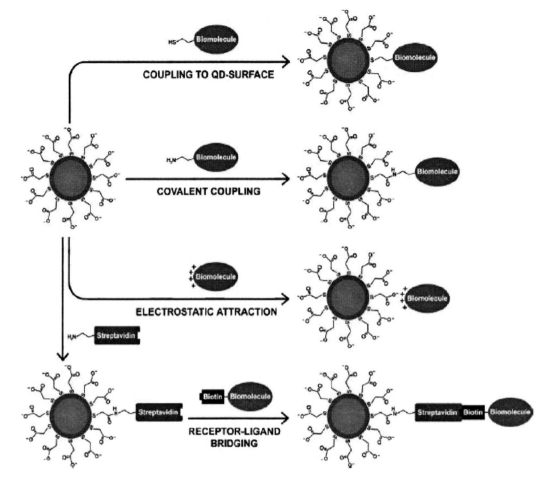

FIGURE 3.2: Schematic representation of common methods to conjugate QDs to biological molecules such as proteins, peptides, nucleic acids, or small organic-molecules

TAT peptides. The image further suggests, from the aggregation of QDs in internal cellular structures, that they are present in endocytotic vesicles [2].

QDs have been used for live imaging of animal organs [6] which are often delivered through the intravenous route to the animals. These studies have successfully demonstrated the ability of QDs to achieve highly specific targeting in animal models. Also such studies reveal that the use of PEGylated QDs could adequately escape the RES providing a unique opportunity for extensive application of QDs in animal models [15]. Fig. 3.5 is the result of a study conducted to evaluate the efficiency of PEG-coated QDs *in vivo* in escaping from the RES and in finding their efficiency for targeted applications. GFE is a peptide having selective binding affinity to the lungs. Injecting mice with red GFE-conjugated QDs showed

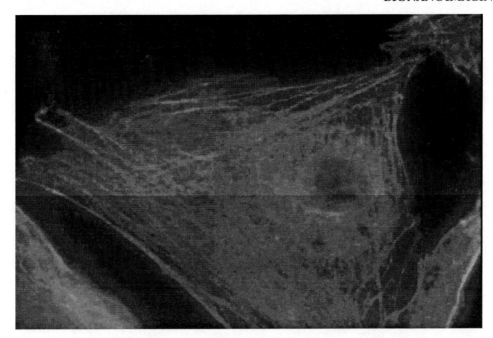

FIGURE 3.3: Immunocytochemical stain of F-actin in fixed fibroblast cells using green quantum dots

preferential aggregation in the lungs, while brain and kidney did not show any QD aggregation, thus proving the high selectivity of targeted QDs [15].

Testing different kinds of QDs in animal models revealed the usability and efficiency of QDs over other luminescent materials. It was notable that PEGylated QDs are readily accepted by the body without resistance from the immune system [15] and also increase the lifetime (of circulation) in the body [6].

F3 is a peptide that selectively binds to the blood vessels and cells of tumor sites. LyP-1 is a peptide that specifically binds to tumor and endothelial cells of tumor lymphatics in certain tumors. QDs conjugated with F3 and LyP-1 peptides were administered via intravenous route in mice having tumor. Fig. 3.6 shows the binding of red F3-QDs binding to the tumor cells and vasculature. While, Fig. 3.7 shows the use how PEGylation can improve the usability of QDs *in vivo*. The LyP-1 QDs initially get trapped in RES and accumulate in liver and spleen, but PEG-coated LyP-1 do not get entrapped in the RES and hence are unseen in spleen and liver [15].

Fig. 3.8 depicts the versatility of the use of QDs in biomedical and biotechnology [7]. The applications of QDs have raised a few concerns, that is being extensively researched currently [16]. Other applications such as live cell single-molecule dynamics study, monitoring of intracellular protein–protein interaction, and disease detection in deeper tissues are possible

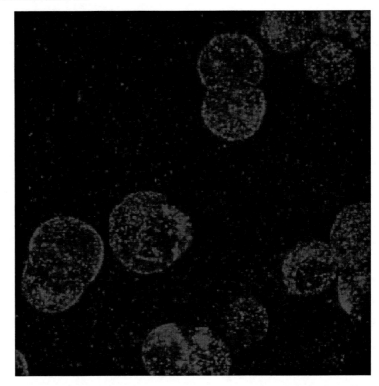

FIGURE 3.4: Cellular uptake of QD-cationic peptide conjugates. Monolayers of living human cancer cells were incubated with red fluorescent (CdSe)ZnS QDs conjugated to TAT peptides. The aggregation of QDs in internal cellular structures is indicative of their presence in endocytotic vesicles

with a higher efficiency in QDs [2, 17]. Also, QDs are even explored in potential applications for cancer therapy. QDs become cytotoxic in the presence of UV; this cytotoxity is explored for the possibility of killing cancer cells [18].

3.2   ULTRASOUND CONTRAST AGENTS

Introduction: Ultrasound is currently a well-established technology enabling real-time imaging of the human body [19–22]. Traditional ultrasound, however, has its own limitation including increase in attenuation with increasing insonating frequency, yielding low resolution of thicker structures, and thus prohibiting deeper scans [23–25]. A possible solution to overcoming the issues of deep scans and achieving improved resolution is the use of contrast agents (CA) for ultrasound imaging [25, 26]. The ultrasound imaging contrast agents (UICA) can be classified into liposomes (μm), polymeric nanosomes, and these are further classified according to the type of ultrasound agent encapsulated in them [27]. Ultrasound imaging (UI) is a noninvasive imaging technique that uses high frequency sound waves to produce images of internal body

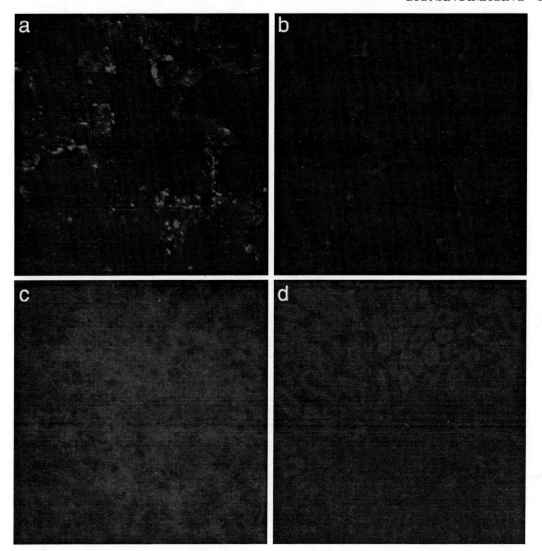

FIGURE 3.5: Red GFE-conjugated QDs injected via intravenous route through a mice tail, (a) red QDs localized in lung tissue, (b) inhibited QDs accumulation owing to coinjected cilastatin, (c) absence of QDs in brain, and (d) absence of QDs in kidney

parts, environment, other biological entities, and organs such as heart, liver, kidneys, fetus, blood vessels, tissues etc. Usually an ultrasound probe which is in contact with the human body (skin) propagates high frequency sound signal into the body which are reflected (echo) back from the internal organs; these signals are reconstructed into images and displayed in a screen. The technique is referred to as UI or ultrasonography (US) and the image obtained is called a sonogram.

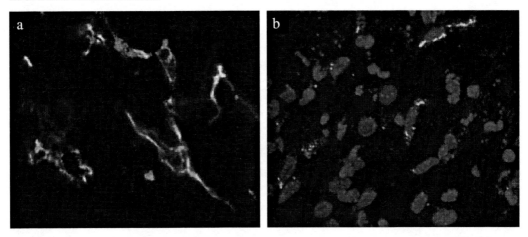

FIGURE 3.6: (a) Red F3 QDs colocalize with blood vessels in the tumors and (b) LyP-1 QDs internalized by tumor cells

Drawbacks of Traditional Ultrasound Imaging: The drawbacks in traditional UI and Doppler include blocking of the US beam by anatomical structures, for instance bones; US beam attenuation or reflection by air and other substances, such as free air, intestinal loops, cirrhotic liver; dense fat pads in the region of organ or site interrogated such as the abdominal fat pad, obese patients, liver enlargement, or hypertrophic muscle bundles; artifacts created by organ movements such as vessels or intestinal loops; and deteriorated patients lacking cooperation or poor patient compliance [24, 25].

Background: Imaging tumors is a prominent part of ultrasound imaging and CA are being developed to improve resolution and diagnostic capability. Typical UICA consist of stabilized gas bubbles. They work on the principle of impedance mismatch with the surrounding tissue, thereby producing better sensitivity and resolution in the image [25, 28]. Traditional contrast agents are mostly micron sized and they are still small enough to move through a capillary. The maximum size that is not barred from entering a capillary is ~8 μm [28]. The biggest challenge, however, is offered by the vasculature of tumors. Tumor tissues have a characteristic angiogenesis that can be easily identified with rich, irregular branching of vasculature that supplies the fast sprouting tissue. The blood vessels observed in and around the tumor site are dense and irregular in size [28].

In ultrasound imaging (UI) the pore size of the tumor vasculature is what determines the maximum diameter of a contrast agent that can successfully penetrate the tumor site. Substantial research results estimate the tumor vasculature pore size between 380 and 780 nm [28]. However, the pore size is characteristic of the type of tumor. The average pore size cutoff for tumor vasculature could be placed at 400 nm. This highlights the very role of

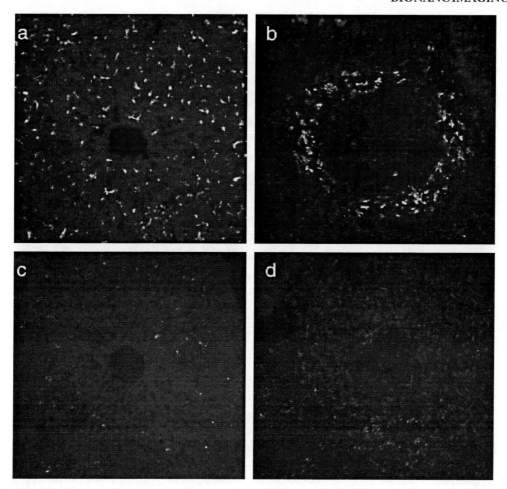

FIGURE 3.7: LyP-1 QDs administered to nude BALB mice with tumor: (a) QDs in liver, (b) QDs in spleen. LyP-1/PEG QDs are not present in (c) liver and (d) spleen

bionanotechnology in creating appropriate nanosize contrast agents to enable imaging of tumors. At present, there exist popular FDA-approved UICA such as Optison®, Definity®, and Imagent® [28].

History of Contrast Agents: The history of CAs dates back to the late1960s when cardiologist Dr. Charles Joiner pioneered the possibility of using microbubbles as echo-enhancing agents [25]. Currently there are more than 29 echocontrast agents in clinical trials throughout the world. They differ noticeably in their chemical composition, action mechanisms, and clinical trial applications [24]. The role of the echocontrast agents (CA) is not limited to improving the acoustic window; they also distend specific organs and fill them with a liquid by causing homogenous attenuation of the ultrasound beam; they displace air-containing intestinal loops;

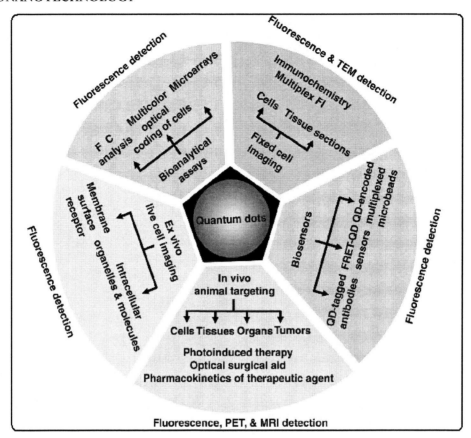

FIGURE 3.8: Versatile applications of QDs in biomedical and biotechnology

they can depict walls, shapes, and contours of cavities both normal and abnormal; they can detect abnormal communications, fistulas, and drainages, as well as evaluate fluid volume in the pleural, pericardial, and peritoneal cavities [24]. Contrast agents find applications in both vascular and extravascular domain.

Most popular vascular CAs include Levovist™ (Germany), BR1 (Italy), and EchoGen® (Abbott, USA). Extravascular CAs include SonoRx™ (Bracco, Italy) and Echovist™ (Schering, Germany) [24]. Vascular CAs are extensively used and are more popular compared to extravascular CAs. Applications for vascular contrast agents in the United States include transcranial color Doppler ultrasound using echocontrast enhancers, contrast echocardiography, neck vessels, liver imaging, vessels in the upper and lower limbs, and focal and diffuse hepatic lesions [24]. Substantial research indicates the higher confidence in diagnostic data with the use of CAs.

Fig. 3.8 shows the image of a US scan of hepatocellular carcinomas (HCC) which is a malignant tumor [24]. In certain cases owing to patient's age, complexity of the developed

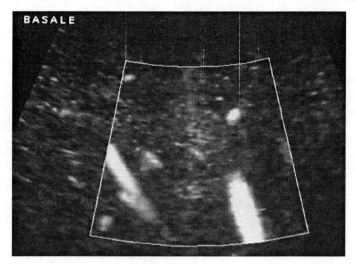

FIGURE 3.8(A): Chemo-embolized hepatocellular carcinoma. Baseline scan, without any CA: no apparent vasculature is seen

tumor lesion resection cannot be performed. For such patients, often nonsurgical/ intervetional procedures are followed, and chemo-embolization is one among the interventional procedures.

No apparent vascularization can be seen in Fig. 3.8 (A). When injected with Levovist, a CA, more color spots and vasculature are noticed as shown in Fig. 3.8 (B) [24]. The prominent

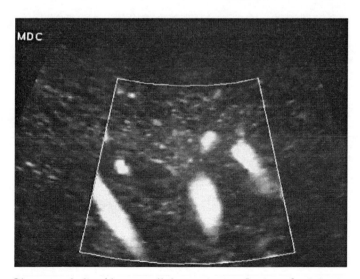

FIGURE 3.8(B): Chemo-embolized hepatocellular carcinoma. Lesion after injection of CA—Levovist: multiple color spots and vessels are seen

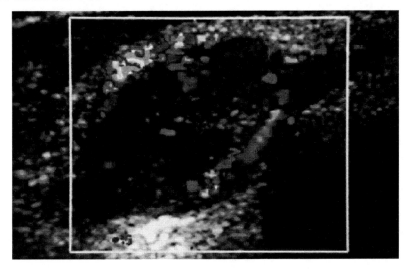

FIGURE 3.9(A): Benign popliteal schwannoma. (a) Before contrast agent injection

role of CAs can further be elucidated with another example. Fig. 3.9 (A) shows an image of a benign popliteal schwannoma condition without any contrast agent. Here no prominent features of the tumor are observed, While the same when injected with Levovist shows a better image of the tumor as in Fig. 3.9 (B) which is a 3D construction of postinjection stage [24].

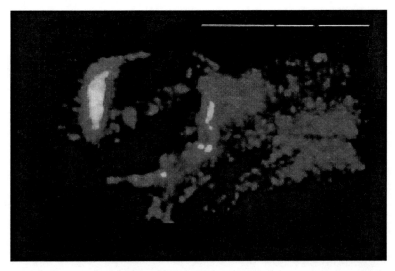

FIGURE 3.9(B): Benign popliteal schwannoma. (b) 3D reconstruction after 2.5 g Levovist^{TM} perfusion at 200 mg:ml

FORMULATION	AVG. GRAY SCALE VALUE (BRIGHTNESS LEVEL)	AVERAGE SIZE (NM)
Inherently echogenic classical Liposomes	115	800
Inherently echogenic sterically stabilized liposomes	109	286
Inherently echogenic (vasoactive intestinal peptides) VIP-sterically stabilized liposomes	119	264

TABLE 3.1: Various Echogenic Liposomes and their Corresponding Size and Gray Scale Values

Table 3.1 shows a list of different kinds of echogenic (echo efficient) liposomes that are employed as contrast agents (CA) in ultrasound imaging [29]. It is interesting to note that the liposomes are much preferred for this purpose as CAs because of the high loading potential they possess in carrying an agent of interest. Usually these liposomes contain gas which is either water soluble such as nitrogen and carbondioxide or water insoluble gases such as perfluorates [29]. Gray scale is a measure of brightness in ultrasound imaging. Table 3.1 shows the gray scale brightness and corresponding nm size of different echogenic liposomal CAs. Gray scale brightness is maintained as the particle size of the liposomes is reduced from 800 to 260 nm.

Among the water-soluble and water-insoluble gas filled liposomes, those with water-insoluble gas are often preferred, probably due to the improved stability and stronger, more long lasting echogenicity because of being water insoluble [27]. Popular water-insoluble CAs include EchoGen or QW3600, Imagent, FSO69, BR 1, NC 100100, and SHU 536 [27].

The most interesting advancement in bionanotechnology would be the design of a CA in the nano domain. A nanosome CA is discussed in detail in this section. The UICA causes significant increase in image resolution through enhanced backscattering signal which is observed from the blood flow. A surfactant-stabilized nano bubble with attractive acoustic properties, better yield, higher stability, longevity of life-time, higher resolution is being developed for application as UICA called ST68-N. This CA is a gas-filled nanosome ranging from 450 to 700 nm in size. This research revolves around the creation of ST68-N as a CA made up of Span 60 and Tween 80. It is filled with perfluorocarbon—PFC (octafluoropropane) gas. *In vitro* test reveals that ST68-N CAs cause *in vitro* enhancement in the UI signals in the range of 27–23 db [28].

The ST68-N contrast bubbles are stable up to 15 min in the body when delivered via the intravenous route. The functioning of the CAs can be well understood with the governing equation–Born's equation that describes the backscattering cross-section σ as being directly proportional to the sixth power of the bubble's radius [28]:

$$\sigma = \frac{4\pi}{9} k^4 r^6 \left[\left(\frac{k_s - k}{k} \right) + \frac{1}{3} \left(\frac{3(\rho_s - \rho)}{2\rho_s + \rho} \right)^2 \right]$$

So the smaller the radius, the lower is the enhancement. However, the diameter is limited to the pore size of the tumor vasculature [28].

Therefore, an optimal function that is able to penetrate tumor vasculature and maximize contrast power needs to be developed. UICA have undoubtedly taken up as the state of art in imaging [26, 30]; the future work in the development of UICAs in the bionano realm will probably focus on the creation of nano CA which are conjugated to biomolecules, thereby rendering them bioactive and site specific in imaging. The creation of CAs with site-specific recognition capability and ability of extravasation from the blood vessels to the tumor site by means of pressure waves and microstreaming [28] caused by ultrasound waves would be a giant leap in the history of UICA. This would enable high resolution imaging of the tumor site itself instead of the vasculature. Bioconjugating these bubbles to biomarkers would yield higher selectivity in imaging the biological interaction *in vivo*.

3.3   MAGNETIC NANOPARTICLES

Introduction: Molecular imaging attempts to visualize quantitative biomolecules or biological processes of interest in living organisms. Such imaging may be noninvasive and possess high targeting and specificity. The contribution of magnetic particles in enhancing molecular imaging increases with the wide clinical application of magnetic resonance imaging. Nanosize magnetic particles enable early disease detection, accurate prognosis, and personalized treatment, monitoring efficacy of a prescribed therapy, or study of cellular interaction in a certain biological environment [31, 32].

The magnetizable particles can independently act as a magnetic probe [32] that can perform an assigned task (bind to an agent). Magnetic contrast agents are dominated by various forms of *iron oxides* especially magnetite/maghemite [33]. Magnetite and maghemite exhibit similar magnetic properties, while maghemite has smaller magnetization saturation. Magnetic saturation is a state at which there is no significant change in magnetic flux density when the magnetization force is increased.

Often the super paramagnetic iron oxide (SPIO) core comes with outer coatings of polysaccharide (mostly dextran) or synthetic polymer coatings which can generally be classified as hydrophilic coatings [34]. Other counterparts of SPIO in the magnetic resonance contrast enhancement domain include gadolinium and cobalt-ferrite particles. The following is a *list of widely used coating materials on SPIO* [31]:

1. Citric, gluconic, oleic
2. Dextran
3. Polycarboxymethyl dextran
4. Polyvinyl alcohol
5. Starches
6. PMMA
7. PLGA
8. PAM
9. PEG
10. PEG-lipid
11. Silane
12. Silica

Based on the overall diameter of a SPIO particle which comprises of the core diameter with the hydrophilic coating, SPIO can be classified into oral SPIO which ranges between 300 nm and 3.5 μm while those ranging between 60 and 150 nm are referred to as standard SPIO or SSPIO. The ultrasmall SPIO (USPIO) refers to particles in the 10–40 nm range. The smallest member of the SPIO group is the monocrystalline iron oxide nanoparticle—MION ranging from 10 to 30 nm. Table 3.2 [31] gives a list of SPIO particles with corresponding size and the level of development.

TABLE 3.2: Commercial SPIO Agents, Corresponding Size, and Developmental Stage

AGENT	SIZE	DEVELOPMENTAL STAGE (CLINICAL TRIAL)
CODE 7228	18–20 nm	Phase II
AMI-227	20–40 nm	Phase III
SHU555A	62 nm	Phase III
AMI-25	80–150 nm	Approved
AMI-121	>300 nm	Approved
OMP	3.5 μm	Approved

Principle of operation: Paramagnetic materials are categorized according to their ability to align their magnetic domains with external magnetic field. This property becomes important in guiding small particles of paramagnetic material to a site of interest in the human body to enhance magnetic resonance by deploying external magnetic field. The magnetic domains of superparamagnetic materials exhibit a random orientation in the absence of an external field but become aligned in response to an external magnetic field. Usually the paramagnetic materials have positive magnetic susceptibility and this enables them to be controlled by external magnetism. The SPIO materials possess very high susceptibility when compared to ordinary paramagnetic material [31]. Magnetic susceptibility is defined as the degree of magnetization of a material owing to an applied magnetic field; higher the susceptibility greater the particles can be magnetized and hence the particular application becomes more efficient.

Coprecipitation and microemulsion techniques are two most common methods to produce SPIO, although methods using ultrasound irradiation, spray, and laser process are described in the literature [31]. Current researches explore the thermal decomposition of precursors (such as iron cupferron—$FeCup_3$, by Alivisatos *et al.*) and a layer-by-layer self-assembly techniques to produce high quality SPIO [31].

The MR contrast enhancement achievable in SPIO could be utilized for [31]:

- Passive Targeting
- Active Targeting
- Cell Tracking
- Magnetic Relaxation Switching

Passive targeting refers to the non-specific cellular uptake of the NPs leading to the particulate accumulation (enhanced retention) in lymph nodes, liver, spleen and macrophage encapsulation [32], and tumor site penetration, enabling better contrast during imaging. Important applications include liver, spleen, or lymph node imaging, as well as general oncological imaging [34, 35]. On the other hand, active targeting relates to the molecule/site specific targeting of SPIO by biomolecular conjugation. The SPIO NPs are functionalized with site-specific biomolecules that render them highly specific and enable to target sites or proteins of interest in the body. Active targeting includes cancer, apoptosis [36], and cardiovascular imaging [31]. Fig. 3.10 [31] shows an application of active targeting of SPIO NPs. Fig. 3.10 is an MRI image of mice with atherosclerosis. The image has been enhanced by the use of active targeted SPIO in the cardiovascular region. The active targeting clearly shows the block in the arterial pathway which is much evident from lack of signal intensity from the site (marked between the red arrows). Another popular *in vivo* application of the SPIO NPs is tracking of

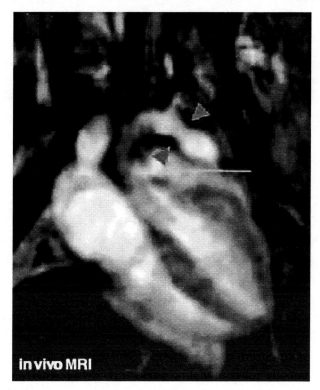

FIGURE 3.10: MRI of mice with atherosclerosis—in the presence of targeted SPIO (yields better contrast and allows detailed imaging)

cellular biodistribution which help us understand how cells migrate and distribute themselves *in vivo* [37].

Another significant application of magnetic NP contrast agents is that of magnetic relaxation switching (MRS)[36] which is being widely used for oligonucleotide, protein and enzyme or enantiomer detection. MRS is a unique property of the SPIO which enables the iron oxide core to diphase the spins of surrounding water molecule protons. This results in the enhancement of T2 (a clarity factor of interest to MR images) or in the enhancement of the spin–spin relaxation time [31, 38]. In either case, MRS improves image clarity multifold mostly due to better contrast with the background. MRS is being used in monitoring and imaging particle–particle interactions such as DNA-DNA, protein–protein, protein–small molecule interactions, or enzyme reactions [38].

REFERENCES

[1] A. P. Alivisatos, "Perspectives on the physical chemistry of semiconductor nanocrystals," *J. Phys. Chem.*, vol. **100**(31), pp. 13226–13239, 1996.

[2] A. Smith, et al., "Engineering luminescent quantum dots for *in vivo* molecular and cellular imaging," *Ann. Biomed. Eng.*, vol. **34**(1), p. 3, 2006.

[3] M. Bruchez, et al., "Semiconductor nanocrystals as fluorescent biological labels," *Science*, vol. **281**(5385), p. 2013, 1998.

[4] R . E. Bailey and S. Nie, Alloyed Semiconductor Quantum Dots: Tuning the Optical Properties without changing the particle size. *J. Am. Chem. Soc.*, vol. **125**(23), pp. 7100–7106, 2003.

[5] J. K. Jaiswal, et al., Long-term multiple color imaging of live cells using quantum dot bioconjugates. *Nat. Biotechnol.*, vol. **21**(1), p. 47, 2003.

[6] B. Ballou, et al., Noninvasive imaging of quantum dots in mice. *Bioconjug. Chem.*, vol. **15**(1), p. 79.

[7] X. Michalet, et al., Quantum dots for live cells, in vivo imaging, and diagnostics. *Science*, vol. **307**(5709), pp. 538–544, 2005.

[8] J. K. Jaiswal, et al., Use of quantum dots for live cell imaging. *Nat Meth.*, vol. **1**(1), p. 73, 2004.

[9] B. O. Dabbousi, et al., (CdSe)ZnS core-shell quantum dots: synthesis and characterization of a size series of highly luminescent nanocrystallites. *J. Phys. Chem. B*, vol. **101**(46), p. 9463, 1997.

[10] W. C. Chan, et al., Quantum dot bioconjugates for ultrasensitive nonisotopic detection. *Science*, vol. **281**(5385), pp. 2016–2018, 1998.

[11] A. L. Efros, and A. L. Efros, Interband absorption of light in a semiconductor sphere. *Sov. Phys. Semicond.*, vol. **16**, pp. 772–774, 1982.

[12] A. I. Ekimov, A. L. Efros, and A. A. Onushchenko, Quantum size effect in semiconductor microcrystals. *Solid State Commun.*, vol. **56**(11), pp. 921–924, 1985.

[13] A. I. Ekimov, and A. A. Onushchenko, Quantum size effect in the optical spectra of semiconductor microcrystals. *Sov. Phys., Semicond.* (English translation of Fizika i Tekhnika Poluprovodnikov), vol. **16**(7), p. 775, 1982.

[14] M. Goulian, and S. M. Simon, Tracking single proteins within cells. *Biophys. J.*, vol. **79**(4), p. 2188, 2000.

[15] M. E. Akerman, et al., Nanocrystal targeting in vivo. *Proc. Natl. Acad. Sci.*, vol. **99**(20), pp. 12617–12621, 2002.

[16] J. K. Jaiswal, and S. M. Simon, Potentials and pitfalls of fluorescent quantum dots for biological imaging. *Trends Cell Biol.*, vol. **14**(9), p. 497, 2004.

[17] Y. T. Lim, et al., Selection of quantum dot wavelengths for biomedical assays and imaging. *Mol. Imaging*, vol. **2**(1), p. 50.

[18] R. Bakalova, et al., Quantum dots as photosensitizers? *Nat. Biotech.*, vol. **22**(11), p. 1360, 2004.

[19] R. Campani, et al., The latest in ultrasound: three-dimensional imaging. Part II. *Eur. J. Radiol.*, vol. **27** (Supplement 2), p. S183, 1998.

[20] F. Candiani, The latest in ultrasound: three-dimensional imaging. Part 1. *Eur. J. Radiol.*, vol. **27** (Supplement 2), p. S179, 1998.

[21] C. Martinoli, et al., Power Doppler sonography: clinical applications. *Eur. J. Radiol.*, vol. **27** (Supplement 2), p. S133, 1998.

[22] M. Bazzocchi, et al., Transcranial Doppler: state of the art. *Eur. J. Radiol.*, vol. **27** (Supplement 2), p. S141, 1998.

[23] J. Langholz, et al., Contrast enhancement in leg vessels. *Clin. Radiol.*, vol. **51** (Supplement 1), pp. 31–34, 1996.

[24] R. Campani, et al., Contrast enhancing agents in ultrasonography: clinical applications. *Eur. J. Radiol.*, vol. **27** (Supplement 2), p. S161, 1998.

[25] F. Calliada, et al., Ultrasound contrast agents: basic principles. *Eur. J. Radiol.*, vol. **27** (Supplement 2), p. S157, 1998.

[26] D. Cosgrove, Ultrasound contrast agents: an overview. *Eur. J. Radiol.*, vol. **60**(3), pp. 334–330, 2006.

[27] G. Maresca, et al., New prospects for ultrasound contrast agents. *Eur. J. Radiol.*, vol. **27** (Supplement 2), p. S171, 1998.

[28] B. E. Oeffinger, and M. A. Wheatley, Development and characterization of a nano-scale contrast agent. *Ultrasonics*, vol. **42**(1–9), p. 343, 2004.

[29] S. Dagar, et al., "Liposomes in Ultrasound and Gamma Scintigraphic Imaging," *Methods in Enzymology*. **373**, pp. 198–214, 2000 doi:10.1016/S0076-6879(03)73013-4.

[30] M. B. Nielsen, and N. Bang, Contrast enhanced ultrasound in liver imaging. *Eur. J. Radiol.* vol. **51** (Supplement 1), p. S3, 2004.

[31] D. Thorek, et al., Superparamagnetic iron oxide nanoparticle probes for molecular imaging. *Ann. Biomed. Eng.* vol. **34**(1), p. 23, 2006.

[32] W. J. Rogers, and P. Basu, Factors regulating macrophage endocytosis of nanoparticles: implications for targeted magnetic resonance plaque imaging. *Atherosclerosis*, vol. **178**(1), p. 67, 2005.

[33] Z. G. Forbes, Magnetizable implants for targeted drug delivery, in *School of Biomedical Engineering, Science and Health Systems*. Philadelphia: Drexel University, p. 139, 2005.

[34] A. Tanimoto, and S. Kuribayashi, "Application of superparamagnetic iron oxide to imaging of hepatocellular carcinoma," *Eur. J. Radiol.*, vol. **58**(2), p. 200, 2006.

[35] J.-K. Hsiao, et al., Labelling of cultured macrophages with novel magnetic nanoparticles. *J. Magn. Magn. Mater.*, vol. **304**(1), p. e4, 2006.

[36] M. Brauer, In vivo monitoring of apoptosis. Prog. Neuro-Psychopharmacol. *Biol. Psychiatr.*, vol. **27**(2), p. 323, 2003.

[37]   A. M. Morawski, G. A. Lanza, and S. A. Wickline, Targeted contrast agents for magnetic resonance imaging and ultrasound. *Curr. Opin. Biotechnol.*, vol. **16**(1), p. 89, 2005.

[38]   J. M. Perez, et al., Magnetic relaxation switches capable of sensing molecular interactions. *Nat. Biotech.*, vol. **20**(8), p. 816, 2002.

CHAPTER 4

Successful Applications of Bionanotechnology

INTRODUCTION

The need to diagnose diseases and medical conditions at an early stage has increased. This is well in accordance with the saying: *prevention is better than cure*. Hence, the earlier we diagnose a condition, the better we stand a chance to prevent a serious condition. New technologies are needed to speed the diagnostic processes and help the scientists and clinicians in the initiation of targeted treatments and in the follow up of treatment responses. An important milestone in this process has been the advances made by researchers in biochemistry, immunology, and drug discovery fields in the identification of molecular signatures of malignancy and cancer, using complicated and cumbersome wet laboratory techniques. The objective now is to exploit those initial accomplishments and combining them with available new technologies to identify the earliest signatures of deadly conditions such as malignancies and cancer. Such developments shall allow us to provide immediate and specific intervention and monitor the progress before it cascades into chronic inflammation and malignancy. The fulfillment of this objective requires the development of technologies of 1–100 nm size which display unique mechanical, electrical, chemical, and optical properties and can assist in visualizing or sensing interactions with receptors, cytoskeleton, specific organelles, and nuclear components within the cells. It would be very rewarding to us when many of these technologies can migrate into monitoring the disease condition through non-invasive methods *in vivo* in a physically undisturbed state, thus minimizing the influence of artifacts induced by physical methods while securing biological samples.

The integration of nanotechnology with biology and medicine has given birth to a new field of science called "Nanomedicine." The ultimate goal of nanomedicine is to develop well-engineered nanotools for the prevention, diagnosis, and treatment of many diseases. In the past decade, extraordinary growth in nanotechnology has brought us closer to be able to vividly visualize molecular and cellular structures. These technologies are beginning to assist us in our ability to differentiate between normal and abnormal cells and to detect and quantify minute amounts of signature molecules produced by these cells. Most of these represent real-time measurements and their dynamic relationship to other structures in the damaged area and also to repair damaged tissues. Novel pharmaceutical preparations have been developed to fabricate nanovehicles to deliver drugs, proteins and genes, contrast enhancement agents for imaging, and hyperthermia agents to kill cancer cells. Several of these inventions have already transitioned into basic medical research and clinical applications. Because of this, several social, ethical, legal, and environmental issues have emerged. Thus, regulatory and educational strategy needs to be developed for the society to gain benefit from these discoveries. The focus of this chapter is to provide an overview of the state-of-the-art in nanotechnology focusing on to its successful application in medicine and allied fields.

4.1   NANOSTRUCTURES AND NANOSYSTEMS

Nanotechnology finding applications in the world of medicine encompasses a wide range of tools and techniques that could efficiently be used as drug delivery platforms, better contrast agents in imaging, chip-based biolabs (MEMS/NEMS), and nanoscale probes able to track cell movements and manipulate molecules [1]. These tools and techniques comprise of combinations of multifunctional nanostructures through cross-disciplinary interactions which would further enhance our diagnostic and therapeutic capabilities, enabling us to monitor intra/extracellular events in diagnostics and therapy.

Evolving avenues of bionanotechnology may impact diagnosis to such an extent that it could facilitate early detection of inflammation, prevention and early detection of cancer including several other diverse technological innovations. The newer avenues would include, but are not limited to bio-mimicking self-assembling peptide systems which serve as building blocks to produce nucleotides, peptides, and phospholipids that support cell proliferation and differentiation and give insights into protein–protein interactions [2].

The microchip drug-release systems, micromachining hollow needles, and two-dimensional needle arrays from single crystal silicon for painless drug infusion, intracellular injections, microsurgeries, and needle-stick blood diagnosis form another group of tools which classify under therapeutic applications [3, 4]. All these developments could one day transform into elements of personalized treatments [5].

Let us recall that the creation, control, and use of structures, devices, and systems with a length scale of 1–100 nm is the domain of nanotechnology and bionanotechnology deals with the diagnostic, therapeutic, and clinical applications of nanotechnology in bioscience, biomedical, and any subunit of Health Care for that matter. Macromolecular structures such as dendrimers and liposomes at the nanoscale are also considered valid nanotools [6, 7]. The application of various nanotools in many areas of medicine is depicted in Fig. 4.1. The list of this figure is by no means exhaustive as nanotechnology continues to grow with newer technologies

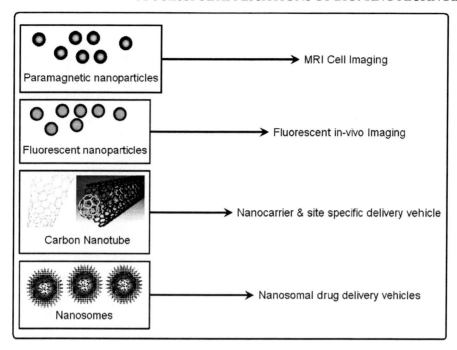

FIGURE 4.1: Bionano tools in Medical applications. [Courtesy of Vishal Kamat and Dr. Papazoglou—Drexel University, Poster Presentation, Biosensors REU Conference, June 2006, Philadelphia, PA.]

emerging each day as we speak. In the following section of this chapter we discuss various capable nanosystems and nanostructures having potential contribution to Health Care.

4.1.1 Nanopore Technology

The biomolecular-nanopore detection technology was first developed to rapidly discriminate between nearly identical strands of DNA thereby replacing the tedious process of running billions of copies of DNA through sequencing machines and thus minimize errors and save time [8]. In this technology single molecules of DNA are drawn through 1–2 nm in size pores that serve as a sensitive detector. The detection system through its electronic signature process can sequence more than one base pair per millisecond. This technology has the potential to detect DNA polyploidy, and DNA mutations.

4.1.2 Nano Self-Assembling Systems

This field involves the feat of biomimetics, dealing with mimicking nature and creating biomolecular nanomachines to address various biological problems. Many biological systems use self-assembly as a means to assemble a variety of complex molecules and structures [9]. Numerous manmade self-assembling systems that imitate natural self-assembly of molecules are created to snap together fundamental building blocks of complex polymer molecules that are structured easily and inexpensively on beads, tubes, wires, flat supports, in suspensions, and liposomes. These assemblies can have genetically introduced bio-functionality so that non-specific molecules are repelled from fusing with the cell membrane fusion layers. DNA, lipid bilayers, ATP synthase, peptides, and protein foldings are all target candidates for self-assembly. Liposomes are a classical example of a manmade supramolecular self-assembling structure.

4.1.3 Cantilevers

Nanoscale cantilevers are about 50 μm-wide flexible diving board-like beams which can be coated with antibodies and DNA complementary to a specific protein or a gene. When molecules come in contact with these substrates coated on the surface of cantilevers, they bind to the substrate and make the cantilevers resonate or bend as a result of this binding event [10]. This bending deflection is proportional to the strength of binding thus making it a quantitative technique. Multiple cantilevers could be used simultaneously to differentiate between bound and unbound molecules. Likewise, multiple antibodies could be used in the same reaction set-up to quantify several markers at a time. An important advantage of this technique is that there is no need to add fluorescent tags to detect and quantify the molecule. Any biological sample containing biomolecules of interest can be tested. Nanoscale cantilevers, constructed as a part of a larger diagnostic device, can perform rapid and sensitive detection of inflammation, procancer molecules, etc. and evaluate how various drugs bind to their targets at a concentration 20 times lower than clinical threshold. A classical example of one of the most successful technologies that evolved out of cantilevers is the atomic force microscopy (AFM) and other scanning probe microscopic (SPM) techniques.

4.1.4 Nanoarrays

Bioassays which are integral part of biotechnology industries as well as associated researches are often cumbersome and error prone. The need for easy and accurate means of conducting the bioassays is an essential requirement. Recent explosive development in the field of microfluidics, biotechnology, and functional genomics has resulted in the miniaturization of these bio-analytical assays to micron scales for routine and throughput screening [11]. These assays could widely be used in genomics, proteomics, and other bioscience analysis. Their application to proteomics still requires refinement since replication of proteins as opposed to DNA is yet to be fully realized. Efforts are underway to further miniature microarrays, which are still used for analyzing proteins. These include fabrication of AFM-based (atomic force microscope) Dip pen nanolithography (DPN) that could probe complex mixtures of proteins, sense reactions involving the protein features and antigens in complex solutions, and study the details of cellular adhesion at the submicron scale. Protein nanoarrays Generated by Dip-Pen Nanolithography are emerging [12] and sooner would evolve into a much power tool in biotechnology. The development of miniaturization techniques like DPN would enable the design of nanoarrays that can detect biological entities on a single-particle level in a timely and cost-efficient manner; also it would profile new diagnostic biomarkers at a detection level much beyond our imagination.

4.2 NANOPARTICLES

Particles in the nano domain could generally be called as nanoparticles. Mostly these are spherical particles with specific properties that allow their detection, analysis, and quantification in a more efficient way. Exhibiting various physical and optical properties, the nanoparticles combine with biomolecules, drugs, and other reagents becoming nanoprobes. For instance, iron oxide nanoparticles exhibit super paramagnetic properties [13] while gold nanoparticles possess specific optical absorption properties depending on their size [14]. It is important to note that particles made from the same materials but of micron dimensions do not exhibit such unique optical or magnetic properties [15]. One can thus combine the immense surface to volume ratio of these nanostructures to deliver higher loads of compounds encapsulated or linked to their surface, while their presence can be measured due to their characteristic magnetic or optical properties. In the following section let us examine various successful applications unique to the nano realm.

4.2.1 Quantum Dots (QDs)

Quantum dots abbreviated as QDs are tiny light-emitting particles on the nanometer scale. They are emerging as a new class of biological probes (in the imaging field) which could replace traditional organic dyes and fluorescent proteins. The fundamental benefit of using quantum dots is their high quantum yield and strong emission intensity. The emission spectrum of QDs is a function of the particle size and hence by varying particle size quantum dots can emit from visible to infrared wavelengths [16]. Let us recall the definition and significance of the Bohr's radius and its relevance to quantum energy from *Chapter 1*.

The QDs can be excited by UV light and emit light, according to their size from the visible to infrared wavelengths. Their broad excitation spectrum and narrow emission spectrum with little or no spectral overlap makes them attractive for high resolution imaging of multiple species at the same time without the need for complex optics and data acquisition systems. QDs offer higher signal-to-noise ratios compared to traditional fluorochromes (fluopores). The high sensitivity of the QDs allows accurate detection even in the presence of strong auto-fluorescent signals encountered during *in vivo* imaging [17, 18]. Their excellent resistance to photobleaching enable for long-term monitoring of biological phenomena, critical in live cell imaging and thick tissue specimens. Already QDs are finding increasing use in live cell imaging, by themselves or as FRET donors combined with traditional fluorochromes, *in vitro* assays, and live animal imaging for cancer and tumor diagnostics. Further, they are used in multimodal applications as contrast agents in bioimaging, microarrays, FACS analysis, and monitor pharmacokinetics of therapeutic agents and in multicolor optical coding for high throughput screening [19].

Limitations of quantum dots can arise from the stability of the core shell structure. Most commercially available materials comprise a core of CdSe and a shell of ZnS. In order to render this inorganic structure hydrophilic, amphiphilic polymers are used to cap the shell layer and provide reactive sites for further linking to proteins. It is therefore the stability of this layer that controls aggregation of quantum dots, as well as possible release of core materials (Cd ions) to the surrounding which may result in toxicity [20]. This has limited the immediate clinical use of quantum dots, but has focused applications to animal testing and *in vitro* assay developments. Simon and colleagues [21] did not notice any cellular toxicity even under selection pressure when they used QDs to track metastatic tumor cell extravasations in an animal model. Quantum dots can have immediate applications in oncologic surgery if the safety profile can be established for humans [22]. However, toxicity to humans is still being debated. Further research is needed before we move forward toward widespread use of quantum dots in biological systems [23]. Another reported problem is the blinking property of the QDs. Quantum dots tend to blink at the single dot level and hence present some limitation in absolute fluorescence quantification. However, when used for imaging of biomarkers this property doesn't affect much as there are hundreds or thousands of quantum dots in a sample to allow proper averaging. More fundamentals, synthesis, conjugation techniques, and applications of the QDs were dealt in *Chapter 3*.

4.2.2 Paramagnetic Iron Oxide Crystals

Paramagnetic iron oxide nanoparticles are a new class of magnetic contrast agents that are finding increasing applications in the field of diagnostic and molecular imaging based on magnetic resonance (MR) [13]. Traditional MR imaging agents rely on the interaction of the proton density, i.e., water molecules and the magnetic properties of the tissue. These paramagnetic agents accelerate the rate of relaxation of protons in the longitudinal direction resulting in bright images and hence are highly dependent on water molecules. However, the super paramagnetic iron oxide nanoparticles by the virtue of their nanoscale properties disturb the magnetic field independent of their environment and hence are not dependent on the presence of water molecules. They are also called negative enhancers [24] as they act as negative contrast agents and appear dark where they are sequestered. The traditional MR agents such as gadolinium–diethylenetriamine penta-acetic acid (DTPA) enhance the signal from the vascular compartments and are nonspecific, whereas the nanoparticle-based contrast agents impact the MR signal from tissues and cells. The gadolinium-based neutron capture therapy has several advantages including more efficient tumor killing effects and the potential for simultaneous MR imaging to assess response. Fokumori and colleagues [25] utilized gadolinium incorporated cationic polymer chitosan nanoparticles that resulted in efficient cellular uptake and demonstrated significant *in vitro* tumoricidal effect at relatively low concentrations.

The superoxide paramagnetic crystals when used in combination with QDs provide additional information of the specific molecular targets for imaging [26].

The advantage of these contrast agents lies in their ability to get sequestered anywhere within a support matrix and still generate a contrast whereas the traditional MR agents need water in their vicinity to generate contrast. These nanoparticles can be used for both passive and active targeting. Because of the small size of these particles, tissue macrophages readily uptake these agents and hence it is possible to image liver, spleen, lymph nodes, and lungs; also they have been able to distinguish between the normal and tumor-bearing lymphatic nodes [27, 28]. These nanoparticles may also distinguish very small metastases (less than 2 mm in diameter) within normal lymph nodes, a size well below the detection limit of the most sensitive imaging techniques such as positron-emission tomography (PET) available today. Metal nanoshells can serve as strong near infrared (NIR) absorbers. This property has been exploited to provide targeted thermal therapy selective to tumor cells without damaging normal tissue using gold nanoshells [29].

In addition, it is also possible to functionalize these nanoparticles using a wide variety of ligands, antibodies, peptides, aptamers, drugs etc. to achieve site-specific or biomarker-specific targeting. This is an added advantage since traditional paramagnetic formulations are difficult to conjugate to antibodies and even when conjugated owing to the small number of cellular receptors, the signal intensity is not sufficient for accurate imaging. The iron oxide nanoparticles find applications as contrast agents for the imaging of cancer, brain inflammation, arthritis, and atherosclerotic plaques. Cells loaded with iron oxide nanoparticles have shown that these particles are nontoxic and are cleared from the cell after 5–8 divisions. Lewin *et al.* [30] labeled stem cells with iron oxide particles using HIV TAT peptide and injected them systemically. The labeled stem cells homed on to the bone marrow and the labeled stem cells didn't cause any impairment. However, due to the small size of these particles a long time is required (up to 24 h) to clear them from the organs and blood to reduce background signals. Thus, MR imaging with the use of super paramagnetic iron oxide particles may result in improved sensitivity and selectivity and may assist to diagnose tumors at the earliest stages of malignancy or metastasis. To have a grasp of insight of iron nano-particles, a thorough substance was presented in *Chapter 3*.

4.2.3 Dendrimers

Dendrimers are a new class of hyper-branched polymer macromolcules that radiate from a central core with structural symmetry. They could vary in shape, size, surface, flexibility, and topography and thus enable fabrication of functional nanoscale materials having unique properties [31, 32]. Dendrimers could be used in the development of antiviral drugs, tissue repair scaffolds, and targeted carriers of chemotherapeutics. Commercially certain dendrimers are now being used as immuno-diagnostic agents and gene transfection vectors. Dendrimers complexed with gadolinium III ions (gadomer-17) are being tested (phase I clinical trial) for magnetic resonance imaging angiography [33], further extending its frontiers.

4.2.4   Carbon Nanotubes

Carbon nanotubes also referred to as "buckytube" or "buckyballs" are a member of the fullerene (C_{60}) structural family that show increasingly potential use in many biological applications. They could be cylindrical (nanotubes), spherical (buckyballs), or branched (fullerenes). Nanotubes could broadly be divided into single-walled nanotubes (SWNT) and multiwalled nanotubes (MWNT). Having adequate characteristics of a "drug-vehicle", the carbon nanotubes are used in drug delivery and cancer therapy significantly backed up by their transporting capabilities achieved via suitable functionalization chemistry and their intrinsic optical properties. Proper surface functionalization is necessary to make carbon nanotubes biocompatible. In one of the recent applications, SWNTs have been used to transport DNA inside living cells [34]. Intracellular protein transport has also been accomplished [35] though they are suspected to provoke severe immune responses. Most SWNTs have diameters as close to 1 nm, with a tube length that could be several thousands times larger. SWNTs with length up to orders of centimeters have been produced [36]. Single-walled nanotubes are a very important class of carbon nanotubes because they exhibit unique electric properties unlike the multi-walled carbon nanotube (MWNT) variants. On the other hand, multi-walled carbon nanotubes fabricated as multiple concentric nanotubes precisely nested within one another can be used for perfect linear or rotational bearing. Technology has now advanced into merging these MWNTs with magnetic nanomaterials like magnetite, which can be functionalized and open newer venues of CNT-associated magnetic applications.

Gado-fullerenes (gadolinium + fullerenes) offer the ability to concentrate more gadolinium at the site of disease (interest), than traditional Gd-DTPA. This is the result of the shielding that the carbon structure provides and its ability to link more gadolinium per conjugate. Gado-fullerenes also take advantage of the gadolinium–water interactions as the gadolinium is along the periphery of the structure and can maintain its interaction with water, which is the basis of traditional proton density MRI. These properties produce a stronger signal which can increase detection sensitivity of even smaller lesions.

Recently there has been further improvement in the aforementioned technology by developing smart bionanotubes which could be manipulated to produce open or closed end nanotubes to encapsulate drugs or genes to deliver them in a particular location in the body

[37]. Thus, possibilities exist for using nanotubes to improve gene sensing, gene separation, drug delivery, and detection of biomarkers for better quality of health care, advanced protection from bioterrorism, and critical progress in other areas of molecular sensing.

4.2.5   Nanosomes and Polymersomes

Phospholipid bilayers exhibiting multifunctional characteristics could be grouped as polymersomes. The polymersomes facilitate the encapsulation of various classes of drugs and diagnostic agents aimed at controlled delivery into cellular and therapeutic targets. Some notable drug delivery strategies utilizing these agents include polymerosomes, hydrogel matrices, nanovesicles/nanofiber mats, and biodegradable nanosomes [38]. They provide as a versatile platform to perform bioscience or biological applications, for instance the biodegradable polymersomes based on polyethylene oxide could be employed as a surface to anchor antibodies or other targeting molecules. Quite recently fluorescent materials have been embedded into these cell-like vesicles [39] to produce near-infrared emissive polymersomes which could be used to locate areas of inflammation and deliver a load of drug to inflammation sites. Interestingly inflammation sites deeper than 1 cm could be imaged with this technique.

To increase the safety and efficacy of gene therapy and genetically derived vaccines, efforts are underway to target DNA complexes into hepatocytes and macrophages. Undoubtedly polymersomes would play a significant role in such applications. Small-sized micelles in the nano domain also classify under nanosomes and are used to develop agents for γ-scintigraphy, magnetic resonance imaging (MRI), and computed tomography (CT)[40]. Liposomes are another integral member of the nanosome family; they are increasingly used in drug delivery applications. A fairly detailed layout on liposomes, their synthesis, and applications is discussed in *Chapter 3* and *Chapter 5*.

A class of polymersomes called polymer nanotubes have been synthesized by directly pulling on the membrane of polymersomes using either optical tweezers or a micropipette [41]. These tubes are unusually long (about 1 cm) and stable enough to maintain their shape indefinitely. The pulled nanotubes are stabilized by subsequent chemical cross-linking. These polymersomes are composed of amphiphilic diblock copolymers consisting of an aqueous core connected to the aqueous interior of the polymersome, less than 100 nm in diameter. The aqueous core of the polymer nanotubes together with their robust character offers opportunities for nanofluidics and other applications in biotechnology especially in the development of nano-hyperdermic syringes [42].

4.3   IN VITRO DIAGNOSTICS

Diagnosis is a key stage in health care; the earlier we diagnose a disease/condition the more effective is the therapy, both from outcomes as well as from a total cost perspective. Bionanotech plays a vital role in the improvement of diagnostic technologies. The development and use of analytical tools in the diagnostic area present immediate benefits to the user. The diagnostic detection techniques involve measuring antibody or antigen-based complexes, enzyme-based reaction rates, or polymerase chain reactions using micro-electro-mechanical systems (MEMS)[43]. Other schemes of scaleable diagnostics include whole cell bacterial sensors and biosensors utilizing aptamers, which are biomimetic synthetic bioreceptors able to complex with proteins, nucleic acids, and drugs. In certain diagnostic methods, the nanoparticles are interfaced with biological molecules such as antigens, antibodies, or chemicals and perform as nanoprobes. Popular nanoparticles employed in diagnostics include quantum dots, metallic nanobeads, silica particles, magnetic beads, carbon nanotubes, optical fibers, nanopores, etc [43].

Similar to the above technologies, nanowires composed of 1–2 nm wide boron-doped silicon wires laid down on a silicon grid can be coated with antigens and provide real-time detection of antibodies (ABs). The AB binding to an immobilized antigen gives a measurable conductance change at AB concentrations less than 10 nM. Detection of single copies of multiple viruses has been accomplished via AB conjugated nanowire field effect transistors (FET)[44].

The dream of optical biopsy is closer to reality with AB functionalized semiconductor nanoparticles (QD's) detected by fluorescence microscopy. Multiplexed assays can be developed since the fluorescence emission of QDs is tunable by changing their size. Outstanding detection sensitivity of antibodies in whole blood (picogram per ml) has been obtained by using gold nanoparticle conjugates [45]. The realization of optical biopsy would revolutionize the medical world.

For detection and characterization purposes classical tools can be used as well as nanobased-methods such as AFM and near-field scanning optical microscopy (NSOM), methods where quantum tunneling plays a key role in amplifying detection capability. This phenomenon is possible due to the nanometer distance between the instrument probe and the surface/specimen under examination. Atomic force microscopy is used to elucidate structures of biomolecules under physiologic conditions [46], determine AB/antigen binding properties [41], image topology of viruses, [47] and image pathologies at the molecular scale [48]. These nano imaging techniques have extraordinary magnification and resolution and can image details of less than 1 nm dimensions.

4.4 MEDICAL APPLICATION OF NANOSYSTEMS AND NANOPARTICLES

It is a longstanding need of the pharmaceutical industry, physicians, and patients to improve pharmaceutical formulations by establishing simpler, less expensive preparations and treatments, while reducing toxicity. This need can be met with the know-how of nanotechnology that has already made breakthrough developments in improved delivery of injectibles, oral formulations, drug device implants, as well as topical and transdermal delivery formulations. Especially in the case of drug delivery to the brain, an *untouchable* region by traditional drug delivery systems, nanotechnology can make the difference. The reason behind the failure of conventional delivery systems in reaching the brain is the blood brain barrier (BBB) composed of tight tissues (*Chapter 3*) making it impervious to outside agents. Nanotechnology has the potential to address and resolve this challenge and make brain a reachable target for drug delivery systems, by combining unique elements of size, surface activity and charge of nanostructures.

Nanosystems and nanoparticles have opened up unforeseen avenues in diagnostics and therapeutics in medicine. The previous treatment strategies in the fields of autoimmune diseases and cancer involved non-targeted treatment options with extensive "collateral damage." Nanodelivery of drugs is envisioned to reduce this collateral damage, extend the drug's availability and effectiveness at the site, and reduce toxicity and cost with a high pay-off load. In this section we present the role of nanotechnology in drug delivery, imaging, and other applications in the biosciences and health care fields. Further details on the background and need of nanotechnology and its potentials were discussed in *Chapter 3*.

4.4.1   Drug Delivery Applications

The focus of this section is to highlight several nanomedical applications, involving biologic nanostructures increasingly used in drug delivery systems. The list of nanostructures include lipid-, silica-, polymer-, fullerene (buckyballs, buckytubes)-based structures such as liposomes, micelles, and other nanoparticle systems.

Liposomal Formulations for Drug Delivery
The definition, fundamentals, and properties of Liposomes were presented in fair detail in *Chapter 3*; the synthetic techniques of liposomes will be discussed in the forthcoming chapter on synthesis techniques of nanoparticles (*Chapter 5*). Liposomes, the vesicles with phospholipid membranes containing hydrophilic substances in their core, often have their properties dictated by the size, lipid composition, surface charge, and method of preparation [49]. Conventional liposomes are short-lived *in vivo* and are rapidly cleared by the reticulo-endothelial system (RES). A novel liposomal formulation with a polyethylene glycol (PEG) coating avoids RES-mediated clearing and is called a *STEALTH liposome,* having properties of long circulation half-life and targeted accumulation in tumor tissues [50].

Liposomes find extensive use in cancer therapy. Some of the major classes of anti-cancer drugs in liposomal formulations are commercially available while others are in late stages of development, and include anthracyclines, camptothecins, platinum derivatives, anti-metabolites and cell-cycle specific drugs such as vincristine and doxorubicin. Liposomal formulations have a demonstrated record of decreased cardiotoxicity as compared to conventional formulations [51]. Current liposomal formulations include pegylated liposomal doxorubicin (Doxil®Orthobiotech, Caelyx®Schering-Plough) non-pegylated doxorubicin (Myocet®Elan Pharma), and liposomal daunorubicin (DaunoXome®, Gilead Sciences).

Liposomal derivatives such as the platinum-derived cisplatin and carboplatin are used in the treatment of head and neck cancers, testicular cancer, lung cancer, and many other malignancies. They have shown significantly reduced toxicity and better pharmacokinetic profiles compared to conventional formulations [52]. Liposomes can conveniently be deployed in passive or active targeting in various cancer applications. In passive targeting, the liposomes can navigate with ease to reach the tumor site due to the high angiogenesis, leaky vasculature, and high permeability of malignant tumors. Passive targeting therefore presents an exceptional opportunity to increase drug concentration at the targeted site by extravasations, thereby reducing toxicity and collateral damage. Active targeting on the other hand depends on c molecular strategies involving monoclonal antibody-liposomal conjugates (referred to as immuno-liposomes) which enable specific tumor cell targeting by antigen identification and drug delivery by internalization of the liposome by tumor cells [53]. The enhanced antitumor activity of anti-HER2 immunoliposomes containing doxorubicin [54] and anti-epidermal growth factor receptor (anti-EGFR) immunoliposomes was demonstrated by increased cytotoxic effect *in vitro*, in tumor cells overexpressing EGFR, and by enhanced efficacy *in vivo* in xenograft models [55].

Liposomal drug delivery also finds good application in treating inflammations; a single dose of PEG-liposome containing glucocorticoids injected in mice (collagen arthritis model) resulted in long lasting joint inflammation reduction as compared to multiple injections required of regular steroids [56]. The role of liposomes in respiratory conditions is also significant, as demonstrated in their performance in asthma therapy [57] and in treating adult respiratory distress syndrome (ARDS), sepsis, radiation lung injury, and emphysema [58] among others. Enhanced drug delivery systems for analgesics [59–61] employ liposomes and are founding increasing clinical acceptance.

4.4.2 Nanoparticles in Molecular Imaging

The basics of nanoparticles and their role in applications and advances of molecular imaging were presented in *Chapter 3* with special emphasis on QDs, MRI, and ultrasound contrast agents. In this chapter, in Sections 4.2.1 and 4.2.2, we discussed QDs and iron oxide nanoparticles which are classical examples of nano-based imaging methods. A variety of nanostructures containing novel contrast agents such as quantum dots, gold nanoparticles, or nanoshells, supramagnetic nanoparticles complexed with biological agents are used to detect malignancy and cancer effectively [62, 63]. There have been efforts to combine drug delivery and imaging; Bankiewicz *et al.* [64] described an integrated strategy to deliver drugs to the brain, where they combined the conventional liposomal drug delivery with an MRI contrast agent (gadoteridol) encapsulated in them. They then used MRI to obtain detailed magnetic resonance images of drug moving through a living primate brain and monitor clinical efficacy. Molecular imaging has now expanded into medical imaging through the use of smart imaging agents for *in vivo* molecular imaging and imaging of animal models [65–67]. A representative example is the use of magnetic nanoparticles conjugated with anti-VCAM-1 antibodies to detect VCAM-1 expression through fluorescence and magnetic resonance on endothelial cells, both *in vivo* and *in vitro* [68].

4.5   SUMMARY AND CONCLUSIONS

Understanding the biological systems, their phenomena at the nanoscale where they operate and their interactions with extraneous nanostructures are the focus of bionanotechnology. Nanomedicine, a much expected outcome of nanotechnology, is a desirable solution to monitor and treat biologic systems in health and disease. This could be accomplished by real-time monitoring of molecular signaling at the cellular and tissue level. The explosion in bionanotechnology research and the associated revolutionary advancements in biomedical applications lay a strong foundation for a customized, personalized, and quantitative medicine in the future.

The present day nanotechnology initiatives include a range of successful and evolving technologies encompassing targeted drug delivery aimed at minimizing side effects, creation of implantable materials as scaffolds for tissue engineering, development of implantable devices, surface modification and designing optimal topology for biomaterial implants, surgical aids, nanorobotics, as well as high throughput drug screening and medical diagnostic imaging. Realizing that the advances possible by nanotechnology will revolutionize medicine, the nanoinitiatives are increasingly funded by government and private sources not only in the United States but also in Europe and the world throughout to develop or to further refine the present technology to provide the beyond imaginable, most sophisticated tools to the physicians and scientists. There will be many technical, regulatory, and legal challenges along the road to implement and realize these technologies. However, there is strong desire and commitment to overcome these challenges and improve the quality of life in a global environment.

REFERENCES

[1] S. M. Moghimi, C. A. H., J. C. Murray, "Nanomedicine: current status and future prospects," *FASEB J.*, **19**(3), pp. 311–330, 2005.

[2] S. Zhang, Emerging biological materials through molecular self-assembly. *Biotechnol. Adv.* **20**, pp. 321–339, 2002.

[3]   D. V. McAllister, M. G. Allen and P. M. R., Microfabricated microneedles for gene and drug delivery. *Ann. Rev. Biomed. Eng.*, **2**, pp. 289–313, 2000.

[4]   D. Sparks and T. Hubbard, Micromachined needles and lancets with design adjustable bevel angles. *J. Micromech. Microeng.*, **14**, pp. 1230–1233, 2004.

[5]   K. K. Jain, Role of nanobiotechnology in developing personalized medicine for cancer. *Technol. Cancer Res. Treat*, **4**(6), pp. 645–650, 2005.

[6]   M. J. Cloninger, Biological applications of dendrimers. *Curr. Opin. Chem. Biol.*, **6**(6), pp. 742–748, 2002.

[7]   M. E. Hayes, et al., Genospheres: self-assembling nucleic acid-lipid nanoparticles suitable for targeted gene delivery. *Gene Ther.*, **13**(7), p. 646, 2005.

[8]   V. W. Wenonah, et al., Rapid discrimination among individual DNA hairpin molecules at single-nucleotide resolution using an ion channel. *Nat. Biotechnol.*, **19**, pp. 248–252, 2001.

[9]   S. Zhang, *Molecular self-assembly In Encyclopedia of Materials: Science & Technology.* Elsevier Science, pp. 5822–5829, 2001, Oxford, UK.

[10] A. Majumdar, Bioassays based on molecular nanomechanics. *Dis. Markers*, **18**, pp. 167–174, 2002.

[11] M. Lynch, et al., Functional protein nanoarrays for biomarker profiling. *Proteomics*, **4**, pp. 1695–1702, 2004.

[12] K. B. Lee, et al., Protein nanoarrays generated by dip-pen nanolithography. *Science*, **295**, pp. 1703–1705, 2002.

[13] M. E. Kooi, et al., Accumulation of ultra-small super paramagnetic particles of iron oxide in human atherosclerotic plaques can be detected by in vivo magnetic resonance imaging. *Circulation*, **107**, pp. 2453–2458, 2003.

[14] J. L. West and N. L. Halas, Applications of nanotechnology to biotechnology. *Curr. Opin. Biotech.*, **11**, pp. 215–217, 2000.

[15] A. Hernando, C. P., and G. M. A., Metallic magnetic nanoparticles. *Sci. World J.*, **5**, pp. 972–1001, 2005.

[16] M. Han, et al., Quantum-dot-tagged microbeads for multiplexed optical coding of biomolecules. *Nat. Biotechnol.*, **19**, pp. 631–635, 2001.

[17] I. L. Medintz, et al., Quantum dot bioconjugates for imaging, labeling and sensing. *Nat. Mater.*, **4**, pp. 435–446, 2005.

[18] P. Mitchell, Turning the spotlight on cellular imaging. *Nat. Biotechnol.*, **19**(11), pp. 1013–1017, 2001.

[19] X. Michalet, et al., Quantum dots for live cells, in vivo imaging, and diagnostics. *Science*, **307**(5709), pp. 538–544, 2005.

[20] J. Lovric, et al., Differences in subcellular distribution and toxicity of green and red emitting CdTe quantum dots. *J. Mol. Med.*, **83**(5), pp. 377–85, 2005.

[21] E. B. Voura, et al., Tracking metastatic tumor cell extravasation with quantum dot nanocrystals and fluorescence emission-scanning microscopy. *Nat. Med.*, **10**(9), pp. 993–998, 2004.

[22] E. G. Soltesz, et al., Sentinel lymph node mapping of the gastrointestinal tract by using invisible light. *Ann. Surg. Oncol.*, **13**, pp. 386–96, 2006.

[23] J. K. Jaiswal and S. M. Simon, Potentials and pitfalls of fluorescent quantum dots for biological imaging. *Trends Cell Biol.*, **14**(9), pp. 497–504, 2004.

[24] J. M. Perez, L. Josephson, and R. Weissleder, Use of magnetic nanoparticles as nanosensors to probe for molecular interactions. *Chembiochem.*, **5**(3), pp. 261–264, 2004.

[25] F. Shikata, et al., In vitro cellular accumulation of gadolinium incorporated into chitosan nanoparticles designed for neutron-capture therapy of cancer. *Eur. J. Pharm. Biopharm.*, **53**(1), pp. 57–63, 2002.

[26] A. J. Bogdanov, et al., Oligomerization of paramagnetic substrates result in signal amplification and can be used for MR imaging of molecular targets. *Mol. Imaging* **1**(1), pp. 16–23, 2002.

[27] Y. Anzai, Superparamagnetic iron oxide nanoparticles: nodal metastases and beyond. *Top. Magn. Reson. Imaging*, **15**(2), pp. 103–111, 2004.

[28] M. G. Harisinghani, et al., Noninvasive detection of clinically occult lymph-node metastases in prostate cancer. *N. Engl. J. Med.*, **348**(25), pp. 2491–2499, 2003.

[29] J. L. West, Nanoshell-mediated near-infrared thermal therapy of tumors under magnetic resonance guidance. *Proc. Natl. Acad. Sci.*, **100**, pp. 13549–13554, 2003.

[30] M. Lewin, et al., Tat peptide-derivatized magnetic nanoparticles allow in vivo tracking and recovery of progenitor cells. *Nat. Biotechnol.*, **18**, pp. 410–414, 2000.

[31] C. C. Lee, et al., Designing dendrimers for biological applications. *Nat. Biotechnol.*, **12**, pp. 1517–26, 2005.

[32] H. Yang, and W. J. Kao, Dendrimers for pharmaceutical and biomedical applications. *J. Biomater. Sci. Polym. Ed.*, **17**, pp. 3–19, 2006.

[33] G. P. Yan, et al., Synthesis and evaluation of gadolinium complexes based on PAMAM as MRI contrast agents. *J. Pharm. Pharmacol.*, **57**(3), pp. 351–357, 2005.

[34] N. W. Kam, Z. Liu, and H. Dai, Carbon nanotubes as intracellular transporters for proteins and DNA: an investigation of the uptake mechanism and pathway. *Angew. Chem. Int. Ed. Engl.*, **45**(4), pp. 577–581, 2006.

[35] N. W. Kam, and H. Dai, Carbon nanotubes as intracellular protein transporters: generality and biological functionality. *J. Am. Chem. Soc.*, **127**(16), pp. 6021–6026, 2005.

[36] H. W. Zhu, et al., Direct synthesis of long single-walled carbon nanotubes strands. *Science*, **296**, p. 884, 2002.

[37] U. Raviv, et al., Cationic liposome–microtubule complexes: pathways to the formation of two-state lipid–protein nanotubes with open or closed ends. *Proc. Natl. Acad. Sci.*, **102**, pp. 11167–11172, 2005.

[38] F. Meng, G. H. Engbers, and J. Feijen, Biodegradable polymersomes as a basis for artificial cells: encapsulation, release and targeting. *J. Control Rel.*, **101**, pp. 187–198, 2005.

[39] P. P. Ghoroghchian, et al., Near-infrared-emissive polymersomes: self-assembled soft matter for in vivo optical imaging. *Proc. Natl. Acad. Sci. USA*, **102**(8), pp. 2922–2927, 2005.

[40] V. P. Torchilin, Recent advances with liposomes as pharmaceutical carriers. *Nat. Rev. Drug Discov*, **4**(2), pp. 145–160, 2005.

[41] E. L. Florin, V. T. Moy, and H. E. Gaub, Adhesion forces between individual ligand-receptor pairs. *Science*, **264**(5157), pp. 415–417, 1994.

[42] J. E. Reiner, et al., Stable and robust polymer nanotubes stretched from polymersomes. *Proc. Natl. Acad. Sci. USA*, **103**(5), pp. 1173–1177, 2006.

[43] T. Kubik, K. Bogunia-Kubik, and M. Sugisaka, Nanotechnology on duty in medical applications. *Curr. Pharm. Biotechnol.*, **6**, pp. 17–33, 2005.

[44] F. Patolsky, et al., Electrical detection of single viruses. *Proc. Natl. Acad. Sci.*, **101**, pp. 14017–14022, 2004.

[45] L. R. Hirsch, N. J. Halas, and J. L. West, Whole-blood immunoassay facilitated by gold nanoshell-conjugate antibodies. *Methods Mol. Biol.*, **303**, pp. 101–111, 2005.

[46] Z. Shao, and Y. Zhang, Biological cryo atomic force microscopy: a brief review. *Ultramicroscopy*, **66**(3–4), pp. 141–152, 1996.

[47] Y. G. Kuznetsov, et al., Atomic force microscopy imaging of retroviruses: human immunodeficiency virus and murine leukemia virus. *Scanning*, **26**(5), pp. 209–216, 2004.

[48] X. Sheng, et al., Adhesion at calcium oxalate crystal surfaces and the effect of urinary constituents. *Proc. Natl. Acad. Sci. USA*, **102**(2), pp. 267–272, 2005.

[49] J. Barauskas, M. Johnson, and E. Tiberg, Self-assembled lipid superstructures: beyond vesicles and liposomes. *Nano Lett.*, **5**(8), pp. 1615–1619, 2005.

[50] L. Cattel, M. Ceruti, and F. Dosio, From conventional to stealth liposomes: a new frontier in cancer chemotherapy. *J. Chemother.*, **16 Suppl** (4), pp. 94–97, 2004.

[51] Y. Matsumura, et al., Reduced cardiotoxicity and comparable efficacy in a phase III trial of pegylated liposomal doxorubicin HCl (CAELYX/Doxil) versus conventional doxorubicin for first-line treatment of metastatic breast cancer. *Ann Oncol.*, **15**(3), pp. 440–449, 2004.

[52] P. K. Working, et al., Comparative intravenous toxicity of cisplatin solution and cisplatin encapsulated in long-circulating, pegylated liposomes in cynomolgus monkeys. *Toxicol Sci.*, **46**(1), pp. 155–165, 1998.

[53] E. Mastrobattista, G. A. Koning, and G. Storm, Immunoliposomes for the targeted delivery of antitumor drugs. *Adv. Drug Deliv. Rev.* 10, **40**(1-2), pp. 103–127, 1999.

[54] J. W. Park, et al., Anti-HER2 immunoliposomes: enhanced efficacy attributable to targeted delivery. *Clin. Cancer Res.*, **8**(4), pp. 1172–1181, 2002.

[55] C. Mamot, et al., Epidermal growth factor receptor (EGFR)-targeted immunoliposomes mediate specific and efficient drug delivery to EGFR- and EGFRvIII-overexpressing tumor cells. *Cancer Res.* 15, **63**(12), pp. 3154–3161, 2003.

[56] J. M. Metselaar, et al., Liposomal targeting of glucocorticoids to synovial lining cells strongly increases therapeutic benefit in collagen type II arthritis. *Ann. Rheum. Dis.*, **63**(4), pp. 348–353, 2004.

[57] K. S. Konduri, et al., Efficacy of liposomal budesonide in experimental asthma. *J. Allergy Clin. Immunol.*, **111**(2), pp. 321–327, 2003.

[58] M. Christofidou-Solomidou, and V. R. Muzykantov, Antioxidant strategies in respiratory medicine. *Treat Respir. Med.*, **5**(1), pp. 47–78, 2006.

[59] W. Huang, et al., Preparation oral liposome-encapsulated recombinant Helicobacter pylori heat shock protein 60 vaccine for prevention of Hp infection. *Di Yi Jun Yi Da Xue Xue Bao.*, **25**(5), pp. 531–534, 2005.

[60] S. Jain, et al., Transdermal delivery of an analgesic agent using elastic liposomes: preparation, characterization and performance evaluation. *Curr. Drug Deliv.*, **2**(3), pp. 223–233, 2005.

[61] A. K. Seth, A. Misra and D. Umrigar, Topical liposomal gel of idoxuridine for the treatment of herpes simplex: pharmaceutical and clinical implications. *Pharm. Dev. Technol.*, **9**(3), pp. 277–89, 2004.

[62] M. E. Ackerman, et al., Nanocrystal imaging in vivo. *Proc. Natl. Acad. Sci.*, **99**, pp. 12167–12621, 2002.

[63] X. Gao, et al., In vivo cancer targeting and imaging with semiconductor quantum dots. *Biotechnology*, **22**(8), pp. 969–976, 2004.

[64] R. Saito, et al., Gadolinium-loaded liposomes allow for real-time magnetic resonance imaging of convection-enhanced delivery in the primate brain. *Exp. Neurol.*, **196**, pp. 381–389, 2005.

[65] A. F. Chatziioannou, PET scanners dedicated to molecular imaging of small animal models. *Mol. Imaging Biol.*, **4**, pp. 47–63, 2002.

[66] S. R. Cherry, In vivo molecular and genomic imaging: new challenges for imaging physics. *Phys. Med. Biol.*, **49**, pp. R13–R48, 2004.

[67] G. Choy, P. Choyke, and S. K. Libutti, Current advances in molecular imaging: non-invasive in vivo bioluminescent and fluorescent optical imaging in cancer research. *Mol Imaging*, **2**, pp. 303–312, 2003.

[68] A. Tsourkas, et al., In vivo imaging of activated endothelium using an anti-VCAM-1 magnetooptical probe. *Bioconjugate Chem.*, **16**, pp. 576–581, 2005.

CHAPTER 5

Synthesis of Gold, Titania, and Zinc Oxide

INTRODUCTION

The small size of nanoparticles (NP) makes them desirable for many biological and biomedical applications. Their size allows them to escape the reticuloendothelial system (RES) and if their surface has been modified for conjugation with biomolecules they become a versatile choice for site-specific drug delivery, imaging, and other diagnostic and therapeutic modalities. NP synthesis addresses the methods and conditions necessary for achieving desirable size and chemistry. In this chapter we discuss several routes and techniques for the synthesis of NPs of gold, titania and zinc oxide, owing to their prevalent use in the health care industry.

5.1 SYNTHESIS OF GOLD

5.1.1 Background

Gold nanoparticles have found extensive biological and biomedical applications and their synthesis is of great interest to the bionanotechnologists. Nanoparticles of gold when functionalized with suitable biomolecules become equipped for targeted applications.

Among the many available synthetic routes [1–9], the most widely used for the synthesis of gold NPs is the Brust method [2], which yields colloidal gold particles of very small dimensions ranging from 1 to 3 nm. The reproducibility of this method makes it the ideal recipe for gold NP synthesis. Thiol functionalization of the gold particle surface enables attachment of biomolecules.

5.1.2 Brust Method of Synthesis of Thiol Derivatized Gold NPs by Biphasic Reduction

This synthesis method involves the growing of nanogold clusters along with simultaneous coating of thiol monolayer around the metallic growths. The governing equation of the Brust method is given in (5.1) and (5.2) respectively. The phase transfer of $AuCl_4^-$ from aqueous to organic phase is a key step and is facilitated by the phase transfer agent TOAB. The addition of

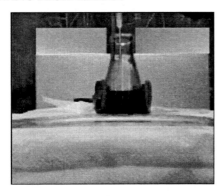 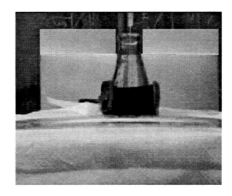

A   B

FIGURE 5.1: Courtesy of Drexel bionanotechnology labs: (A) initial orange color of the aqueous and organic mixture containing $AuCl_4^-$ before adding the reducing agent and (B) dark brown color of the solution after the addition of the reducing agent $NaBH_4$

the reducing agent $NaBH_4$ is marked by a significant color change from orange (before adding) to dark brown (few seconds after the addition) as shown in Fig. 5.1 (A), (B). The reduction has been carried out in the presence of DDT. This technique yields gold nanoparticles of 1–3 nm size. Fig. 5.2 shows the TEM images of the gold NPs obtained.

$$AuCl_4^- (aq) + N(C_8H_{17})_4^+ (C_6H_5Me) \rightarrow N(C_8H_{17})_4^+ AuCl_4^- (C_6H_5Me) \qquad (5.1)$$

$$mAuCl_4^- (C_6H_5Me) \rightarrow 4mCl^- (aq) + nC_{12}H_{25}SH(C_6H_5Me)$$
$$+ 3me^- + (Au_m)(C_{12}H_{25}SH)_n(C_6H_5Me) \quad (5.2)$$

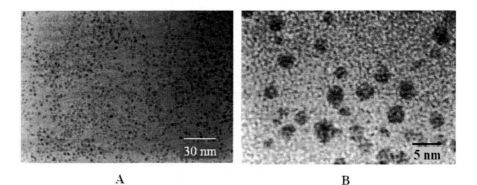

A   B

FIGURE 5.2: TEM images of thiol derivatized gold NPs (A) low magnification and (B) high magnification

Alterations were made to the Brust method and to optimize synthesis of specific particle sizes [1, 8]. Equations (5.3) and (5.4) suggest the possible particle sizes with respect to the chosen molar concentration of the reactants.

$$0.11\,M\,DDT\,(1\,ml) + 0.11\,M\,MPA\,(1\,mL)\ \text{followed by addition of NaBH4.} = 5\,nm$$
$$(5.3)$$

$$0.22\,M\,DDT\,(1\,ml) + 0.22\,M\,MPA\,(1\,mL)\ \text{followed by addition of NaBH4.} = 3\,nm$$
$$(5.4)$$

This approach involves the use of mercaptopropionic acid (MPA) in combination with DDT during reduction [8]. One of the key features of the Brust method is that the final product (Thiol-functionalized gold NPs) is stable for several weeks unlike the usual products which agglomerate over a period of time and eventually collapse from their colloidal assembly.

In the following sections of the chapter, we present a collection of various nano structures of different materials of interest to the biotechnology Industries. These nano structures could be classified on the basis of their size, shape, state, and so on. A general list would include nano tubes, nano colloids, nano rods, nano "branched" rods, nano wires, nanofilms, nano shells, nano spheres, etc.

5.1.3   Gold Colloids
The following TEM image in Fig. 5.3 shows colloidal gold nano-particles of sizes 3–8 nm [8].

5.1.4   Gold Nanofilm
Fig. 5.4 shows the 3D AFM image of ultra-thin (1–15 nm) gold films on glass substrates [3].

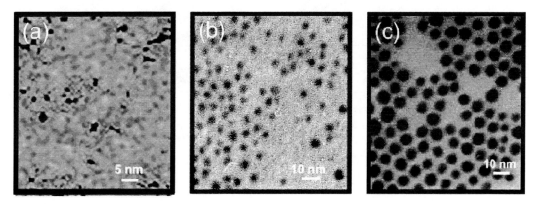

FIGURE 5.3: TEM images of colloidal gold (a) 3 nm, (b) 5 nm, and (c) 8 nm

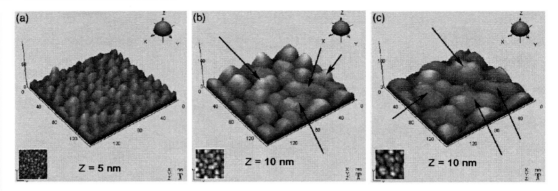

FIGURE 5.4: 3D AFM images (150 × 150 nm^2) of gold thin films (monolayer) (Arrows in the image indicate coalescence)

5.1.5   Gold Nanorods

The TEM images in Fig. 5.5 correspond to gold nano rods of varying aspect ratios, namely 13 and 18 respectively [5].

5.2   SYNTHESIS OF TITANIA NANOSTRUCTURES

5.2.1   Background

Titanium-di-oxide (TiO$_2$-titania), the naturally occurring oxide of titanium, not available in pure form is often synthesized from its ilmenite or leuxocene ores. Among the various forms of TiO$_2$ the rutile, anatase, brookite, and titanium dioxide (B) are the prevalent materials.

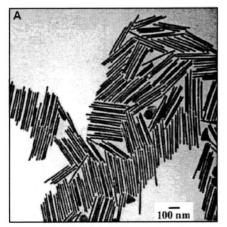
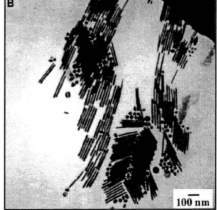

FIGURE 5.5: TEM images of gold nano rods of aspect ratio (A) 18 and (B) 13

Synthesis of titania had always been a subject of interest to the chemical and biochemical industries because titania possesses versatile properties, extensively harnessed by a wide range of industries. Substantial literature asserts the ability of titania to be used as an exemplary catalyst [10–17], finding applications in the decomposition of organic pollutants, in water purification installations, in the paint and polymer industry, the pharmaceutical, and cosmetics industry (UV absorber).

Combining the activity of titania to a particle size in the nanorange expands its capabilities and applications. Its catalytic activity is dependent mainly on the particle size [10, 15]. The smaller the size, the greater is the activity. Earlier researchers mostly focused on the photocatalytic applications of TiO_2 including water purification and pollutant decomposition. More recent studies revealed that metal or semiconductor doped titania has superior photocatalytic activity compared to pure titania [8, 18, 19]. Such results have created renewed interest in developing more efficient methods of TiO_2 synthesis. Synthesis of titania NP can be achieved by various routes, sol-gel, microemulsion, flame oxidation, and others. These can produce titania particles from 4.4 nm to 2300 nm (2.3 µm). For our purpose, we will focus on methods yielding particle sizes from 4 nm to 200 nm.

5.2.2   Solvo-Thermal Synthesis of Titania Nano Crystals

This process involves the synthesis of titania nanoparticles in toluene with an average particle size of 20 nm using titanium isopropoxide (TIP) as the precursor [20].

The wt% ratio of the precursor (TIP) to the solvent (toluene) determines the ultimate particle size. The reaction must be carried out in an inert atmosphere (argon). The nano crystals produced by this method [20] when examined by TEM and XRD revealed an average crystal size of 20 nm. Fig. 5.6 shows the TEM images of titania nanocrystals formed from TIP/toluene solution of various ratios (SPECIFICS). Increase in the amount of the precursor (TIP) used [20] results in corresponding increase in the nano-crystal size. The synthesis details of this method could be referred in Appendix 5.2.2.

5.2.3   Sol-Gel Template Synthesis of Titania Nano Tubes and Rods

A template synthesis method usually comprises of a template into which the desired nanoparticles are formed and grown. Titania nanoparticles produced by the sol-gel method are formed into an alumina template. Several synthesis techniques existed already for the template synthesis of titania [21–24]. This method emerged as the preferred method to produce titania nanoparticles of uniform and controlled particle size yielding nano tubes of various desired thickness and diameters [25].

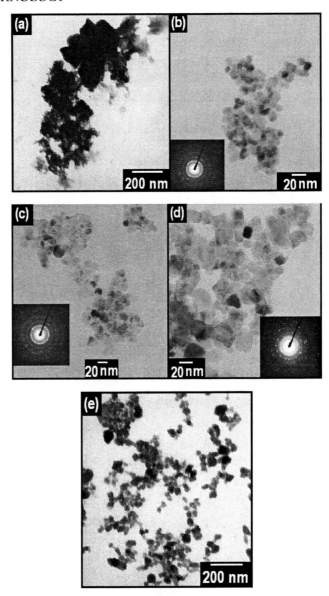

FIGURE 5.6: TEM images of titania nano-crystals formed from TIP/toluene ratio of (a) 5:100, (b) 10:100, (c) 20:100, (d) 30:100, and (e) 40:100 respectively

Table 5.1 shows the particle diameter as a function of the alumina wall thickness, the ratio of reactants and the dipping time. The details of the synthesis are given in Appendix 5.2.3. The TEM images in Figs. 5.7, 5.8, and 5.9 show the wall thickness, diameter, and size of the nano tubes synthesized from various molar concentrations [25].

TABLE 5.1: Relationship Between the Molar Ratios of the Precursor to Other Reactants and the Wall Thickness and Diameter in the Synthesis of the Titania Nano Tubes/Rods.

	MOLAR RATIO OF TI:ACAC: H₂O:ETOH	DIPPING TIME (MIN)	WALL THICKNESS	TUBE DIAMETER (NM)
1.	1 : 2 : 3 : 20	10	50 nm	200
2.	1 : 1 : 3 : 20	10	15–20	10
3.	1 : 1 : 3 : 40	10	–	200–250

In summary, the wall thickness decreases in direct proportions to the concentration of ACAC used. However, the nano tube's dimensions could also be controlled by varying the dipping time [22–24].

5.2.4   Overview of Other Synthesis Methods
A) Sol-gel Synthesis by Ultrasound-irradiation of TiO₂

This technique involves the synthesis of nanosized TiO_2 particles via ultrasonic irradiation [15]. This process is a combination of sol gel synthesis + hydrolysis of titanium isopropoxide and ultrasonication, done by adding to pure water, titanium isopropoxide (TIP). The synthesis details are given in Appendix 5.2.4 A. Using this method, particles' size varying from 5.1 to 21.6 nm with increasing size with increased temperature of calcinations is obtained. TiO_2 of size 14 nm is obtained for the ultrasound irradiated process, while the nonirradiated process yielded particle size of 22 nm [15].

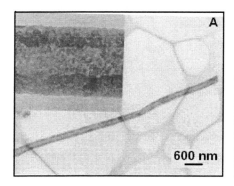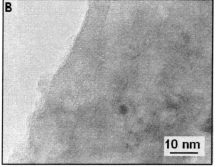

FIGURE 5.7: TEM nano-tubes of 200 nm diameter and 50 nm wall thickness

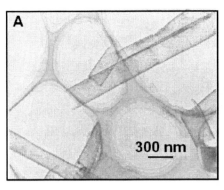
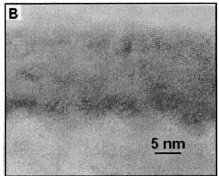

FIGURE 5.8: TEM nano-tubes of 15–20 nm wall thickness

B) Microemulsion-based Synthesis of TiO_2

This method involves the hydrolysis of titanium tetraisopropoxide (TTIP) in W/O microemulsions comprising of water, tween series surfactants of various hydrophobic groups, and cyclohexane. Involving centrifugation at higher rpms, this method yields microemulsion which is dried and later calcined at higher temperatures. This process produces titania nanoparticles varying from 9 through 17 nm [14]. The synthesis details could be referred in Appendix 5.2.4B.

C) Metal/Semiconductor Doped Synthesis of TiO_2

Titania when synthesized by doping with a metal (one or more metals) or a semiconductor resulted in better catalytic activity [8, 19]. The source of excitations is usually visible light or UV rays. Various combinations resulting in different sizes collectively indicated the enhanced catalytic activity to doping of titania. Notable among the doped families are, Ru–Co–Ti, Ti–Au–Co, TiO_2–SiO_2, TiO_2–Ag, and Ti-tungsten doping [8, 11, 18, 19]. Particle size as small as 1.38 nm could be produced by doped synthesis methods [18].

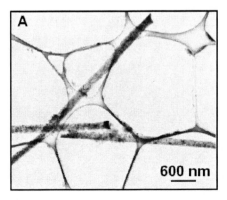
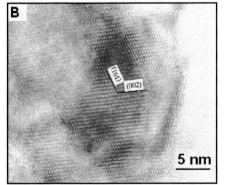

FIGURE 5.9: TEM nano-rods of 200–250 nm diameter

Other notable methods include low temperature synthesis [17], dendrimer protected method [26], etc. Further, the knowledge of optimum conditions designed for the synthesis of titania nanoparticles throw light upon the much needed synthesis expertise [27].

5.3   SYNTHESIS OF ZINC OXIDE

5.3.1   Background

Zinc oxide (ZnO), commonly known as zinc white or calamine, is naturally found as zincite mineral. It is white in color and cubical in structure. Zinc oxide is also associated with its wurtzite structure as shown in Appendix 5.3.2. Ever since the early times of the modern age of science, around early 1960s, ZnO has been a material of industrial significance [28]. For instance, its white color is used in paint industries as a base and it is more transparent than titania—its prevalent counterpart. ZnO processes excellent physical and structural properties; the most notable of them is its pyroelectric and piezoelectric property [28]. Pyroelectric refers to the property of a material to generate electric potential when heated or cooled, while piezoelectricity refers to the property of a material (crystal) to generate voltage when subjected to mechanical stress. The piezoelectric property of ZnO is attributed to its noncentral crystal symmetry. More details of the crystallography of ZnO and its typical growth structures could be referred elsewhere [28].

Yet another interesting fact about ZnO is its semiconductor properties, it has a band gap of 3.37 eV finding applications in optoelectronics. Further, ZnO is known to have contributed to field of sensors, transducers, and catalysts [28]. The increasing know-how of synthesizing ZnO nano-structures and its overwhelming properties show a promising a pathway to achieve breakthrough in optoelectronics, photonics, sensors, transducers, biomedical sciences, etc. The fact that ZnO nano belts have evolved into nano-sensors, nano-cantilevers and field effect transistors (FETs), and nano-resonators adds eminence to its prospective [28].

This section of the Chapter deals with the synthesis aspects of ZnO and the associated parameters of chief interest in the synthesis, emphasizing on one particular method, namely the sublimation (solid-vapor) technique. It involves a high-temperature heating of zinc precursor which facilitates a solid to vapor transfer [28]. Later the vapor is cooled down to be grown into desired pattern and sizes. Using the solid-vapor method a variety of nanostructures such as nano tubes, nano rods, nano combs, nano rings, nano belts, nano helixes, nano springs, nano wires, nano saw, and even nano cages are possible [28]. Undoubtedly, ZnO classifies one of the richest family of nano structures having immense applications [28, 29].

5.3.2   The Solid-Vapor Synthesis of ZnO

As mentioned earlier the synthesis techniques of various nanostructures of ZnO described in this section would deal with the solid-vapor method. The solid-vapor process involves the evaporation of a condensed or powdered material (of interest—ZnO) into its vapor phase which is later allowed to condense under the desired experimental conditions of pressure, temperature, atmosphere, etc. to form the various nanostructures [28].

The solid-vapor method solicits the use of a horizontal tube furnace, the details of which are discussed briefly in Appendix 5.3.1. The key point to be noted in this synthesis technique is that the parameters that dictate the morphology, size, etc. of the product are the temperature, pressure, the atmosphere, the substrate, time of evaporation, and the flux of gas [28, 30–32].

a) Nanorods

The nanorods of ZnO are synthesized by following a vapor-liquid-solid (VLS) approach. This approach involves the use of a *nanorod/wire component* and a *catalyst component,* both subjected to the ideal reaction conditions. All the reactants after undergoing evaporation condense to form the product during which the nanorods grow. Fig. 5.10 shows an SEM image of ZnO nanorods synthesized on an alumina substrate with Au as the catalyst [28]. Compared to gold (Au), tin (Sn) is nevertheless an eligible choice as a catalyst [30]. The use of Sn as a catalyst produces more uniform nanorods [32]. Fig. 5.11 shows the image of aligned nanorods of ZnO grown on a ZnO crystal carried out in the presence of Sn [32]. In these techniques, the choice of the substrate plays a crucial role in the synthesis by governing the consequent morphology of the nanostructures. The synthesis details of the ZnO nanorods could be found elsewhere [28, 30–32].

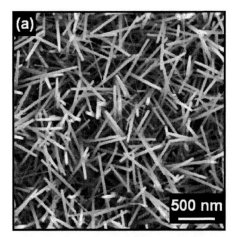 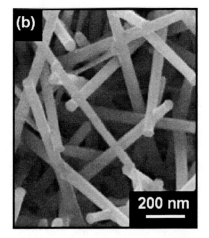

FIGURE 5.10: SEM images of ZnO nano rods synthesized using Au as a catalyst. (a) Small magnification and (b) higher magnification

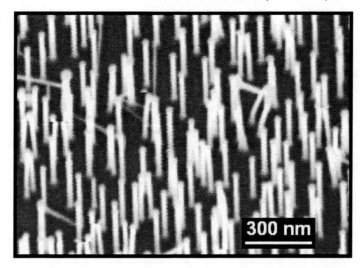

FIGURE 5.11: SEM image of aligned ZnO nanorods/nanowires epitaxially grown on ZnO substrate using Sn as a catalyst

b) Nanobelts

Nanobelts of ZnO are synthesized by mere sublimation of ZnO powders in the absence of a catalyst. The typical structures of the nanobelts range from 50 to 300 nm in width and 10–30 nm in thickness as shown in Fig. 5.12 [33].

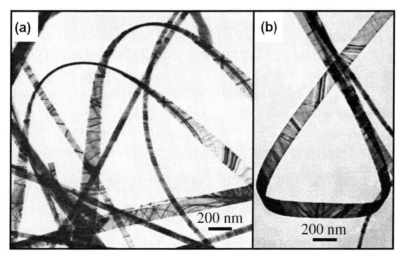

FIGURE 5.12: TEM images of the as-synthesized ZnO nanobelts, showing uniform morphology. (a) Smaller magnification and (b) higher magnification

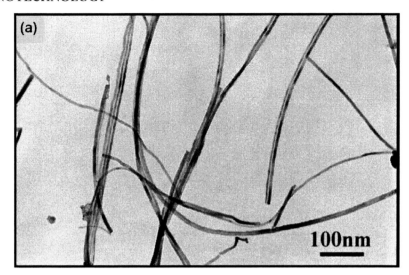

FIGURE 5.13: TEM image of ultrathin nanobelts of ZnO

　　Ultrathin nanobelts could be produced by the use of Sn catalyst which is in the form of a thin film coating of 10 nm on the substrate used. The use of Sn catalyst yields very thin nanobelts of average diameter 5.5 nm, [34] as shown in Fig. 5.13 [34]. More synthesis details on nano belts and ultrathin nanobelts could be referred elsewhere [28, 33–35].

c) Hierarchical Nanostructures
The hierarchical nanostructures comprise of a central axial nanowire surrounded by nanobranches. The hierarchical nanostructures are yet other possible exotic morphologies of the ZnO clan as shown in Fig. 5.14 [36]. The synthesis technique of the hierarchical nanostructures employs the use of Sn catalyst which initiates and leads the growth of the ZnO wires [28, 36]. The entire growth process could broadly be viewed in two stages: the growth of the central axis and that of the surrounding branches. The surrounding nanobranches on the central axis are symmetrical in six directions with a mutual angular displacement of 60° thus giving a more uniform and aesthetic look. The details of the synthesis involved in producing the hierarchical nanostructures could be referred elsewhere [9, 37, 38].

d) Nanocombs and Nanosaws
The growth of nanocombs/sawlike structure as depicted in Fig. 5.15 [36] involves the synthesis procedure as described elsewhere [36, 39]. The synthesis could however be self-catalyzed growth in the absence of catalyst [36]. These immaculate structures are not only limited to ZnO but

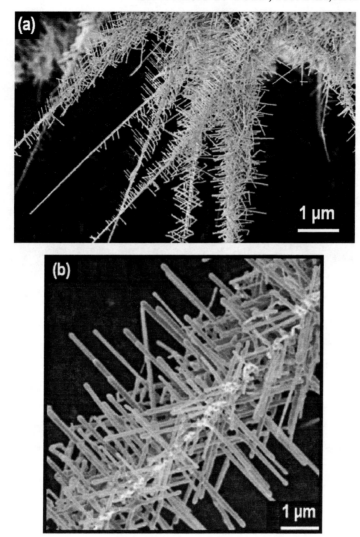

FIGURE 5.14: SEM images of the hierarchical ZnO nanowire junction arrays, (a) smaller magnification and (b) higher magnification

also have been revealed for ZnS [40] and CdSe. Further details on nanocomb synthesis could be referred elsewhere [36, 39–41].

e) Nanorings, Nanospirals, and Nanosprings
It has been demonstrated that In/Li doped ZnO yield polar surfaces in the resulting product [42]. A polar surface [43] dominated nanobelt could be picturized as a capacitor with two parallely charged plates as shown in Fig. 5.16(a) [44]. By the laws of nature, the nanobelt would

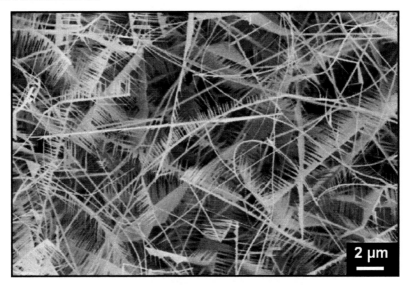

FIGURE 5.15: SEM image of ZnO nanocombs

try to attain a low energy state and hence it could take shape into a ring or a spiral or a spring as shown in Figs. 5.16(b), 5.16(c), and 5.16(d) [44]. Further synthesis details could be referred elsewhere [42, 44, 45]. The thickness of the nanobelts obtained by the doping technique ranges from 5 to 20 nm with an aspect ratio of 1:4; they are extremely tough and flexible [28].

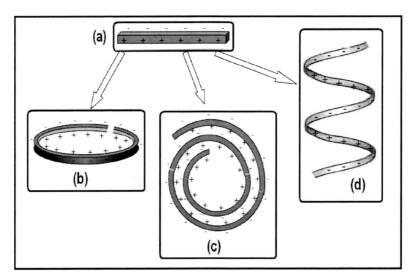

FIGURE 5.16: (a) The model of a polar nanobelt. (b), (c), and (d) are various shapes induced by the polar surface of the ZnO

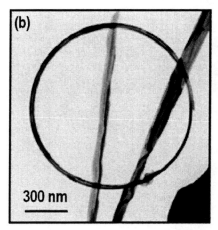

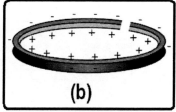

FIGURE 5.16(b): TEM image of a Zno nanoring

f) Nanocantilevers

Cantilevers of small sizes play a crucial role in modern day imaging, especially in scanning probe microscopy (SPM). A classical example would be the AFM. Traditionally the SPMs use Si, Si3N4, or SiC cantilevers of typical size of 100 nm in thickness, 5 um in width, and 50 um in length [28]. A smaller cantilever would allow more precision and details in probing. The potential applications of using carbon nanotubes grown on cantilever tips have already been proven and have been accepted to provide more details in surface morphology of the scanned samples [46]. The possibility of using ZnO nanobelts as AFM cantilevers has also been demonstrated [47]. Given the above situation, it is time of the nano realm to take over SPM and revolutionarize it. The marriage of MEMS/NEMS (micro/nanoelectromechanical systems) and the nano cantilevers would undoubtedly open newer avenues in the development of devices for force, pressure, mass, thermal, biological, and chemical sensors. The smaller the

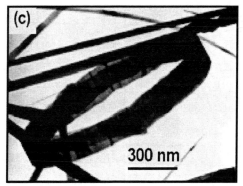

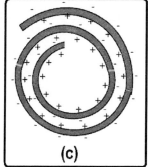

FIGURE 5.16(c): TEM image of a ZnO nanospiral

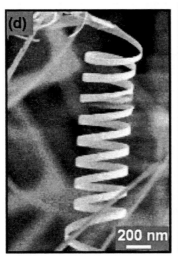
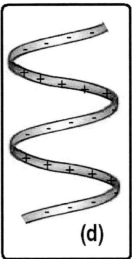

FIGURE 5.16(d): TEM image of a ZnO nanohelix

size the better is the sensitivity of cantilevers. The synthesis details of nanocantilevers could be referred elsewhere [47].

The ZnO cantilevers shown in Fig. 5.17 correspond to various lengths; these cantilevers have been aligned onto a silicon chip [47]. These cantilevers would eventually find applications

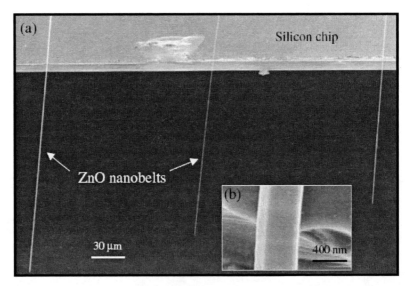

FIGURE 5.17: (a) Nanobelts as ultrasmall nanocantilever arrays aligned on a silicon chip. (b) An enlarged SEM image recorded from the nanobelt cantilever

in SPM, which could be, but not limited to the contact, noncontact, and tapping modes of AFM.

g) Piezoelectric-Nanoactuators and Nanosensors

The AFM measurement of piezoelectric coefficient of ZnO nanobelts reveals that the coefficient d33 of ZnO varies from 14.3 to 27.7 pm/V [48]. This high value suggests the possibility of applications of ZnO nanobelts as nanoactuators and nanosensors. Another interesting application is the development of a ZnO nanorods/wires based hydrogen and ethanol sensor [49].

APPENDIX 5: SYNTHETIC ROUTES FOR NANOPARTICLES
5.1
5.1.1 Brust Method of Synthesis of Thiol Derivatized Gold NPs by Biphasic Reduction

The method of synthesizing thiol derivatized gold NP of 1–3 nm size involving bi-phasic reduction (involving an aqueous to organic phase transfer of gold particles). The following is the list of materials and method of synthesis –

Materials.

1. $HAuCl_4$—hydrogen tetrachloroaurate trihydrate
2. DDT—dodecanethiol
3. TOAB—tetraoctylammonium bromide
4. $NaBH_4$—sodium borohydride
5. Toluene
6. Ethanol

Method. This technique involves the fabrication of thiol-coated gold NPs. An aqueous solution of 25 ml, 30 mmol/L of $HAuCl_4$ is mixed with a solution of 80 ml, 50 mmol/L TOAB in toluene. The mixing is followed by vigorous stirring until there is a phase transfer of $AuCl_4$ d from the aqueous phase to the organic phase. Then 170 mg of DDT is added to the organic phase (containing the $AuCl_4-$). Now, freshly prepared aqueous solution of 25 ml, 0.4 mol/L of $NaBH_4$ is added in minute quantities amidst vigorous stirring (usually delivered through a syringe pump-needle set up). The stirring is continued for over 3 h and then the organic phase containing gold is separated from the aqueous phase [2].

Then, in a rotary evaporator the organic-gold solution is evaporated to 10 ml and mixed with 400 ml of ethanol in order to remove the excess thiol on the surfaces. The resulting solution is subjected to −18°C for 4 h, in dark, yielding a brown precipitate. This precipitate is filtered and later washed with ethanol. The resulting product is dissolved in 10 ml of toluene and precipitated with 400 ml of ethanol. This method provides a simple route of synthesis of gold NPs with thiol functionalization. The TEM images, as shown in Fig. 5.2, reveal the particle size and other interesting features of the thiol functionalized gold NPs. The particle size had maximum distribution between 2 and 2.5 nm and were found between 1 and 3 nm. Also, the synthesized particles were mostly individually and very few were found twinned, unlike other synthesis methods. As a result, this method is much in favor for an ideal choice of gold NP fabrication [2].

5.2
5.2.1   Solvo-Thermal Synthesis of Titania Nano Crystals

This process involves the synthesis of titania nanoparticles in toluene with an average particle size of 20 nm using titanium isopropoxide (TIP) as the precursor [20]. The wt% ratio of the precursor (TIP) to the solvent (toluene) determines the ultimate particle size. The reaction must be carried out in an inert atmosphere (argon).

   Reactants:

   1.   Titanium isopropoxide (Ti(OCH(CH$_3$)$_2$)$_4$ 97%- TIP (Aldrich)
   2.   Anhydrous toluene 99.8% (Aldrich)

Method. TIP and toluene are mixed in the proportions of 5:100, 10:100, 20:100, 30:100, and 40:100, respectively in the presence of argon atmosphere in a glove box. The corresponding wt% of TIP in the organic solution, in the above-mentioned concentrations, are 5%, 9%, 17%, 23%, and 29% respectively. Each of the solutions is mixed vigorously for 3 h by a magnetic stirrer. After stirring, the solutions are transferred into an autoclave (stainless steel autoclave with Teflon lining—capacity of 130 mL and 80% filling) and heated at 250°C at the rate of 4°C/min for 3 h (without stirring). Later the system is cooled down to room temperature. Earlier, the thermal treatment causes the decomposition of TIP into the organic solution and later upon cooling crystallization occurs, producing nano crystals of titania. After cooling the precipitates are separated using a centrifugal separator and dried.

5.2.2   Sol-Gel Template Synthesis of Titania Nano Tubes and Rods

A template synthesis method usually comprises of a template into which the desired nanoparticles are formed and grown. Gold nanoparticles produced by the sol-gel method are formed into an alumina template. Several synthesis techniques existed already for the template synthesis of titania [21–24]. However, most of these earlier methods were inappropriate for industrial production and lacked reliability owing to very short dipping times and also there were issues related to hydration of TIP rendering it milky white and undesired [22–24]. Moreover, these techniques did not study the details and the role of molar concentration in determining the particles size and shape [22–24]. The method described here is more reliable and controllable while having studied the role of molar concentration on particle synthesis in detail [25].

The sol-gel template synthesis technique involves the use of commercially available "Whatman Anopore filters from Fisher" as templates to synthesize the nano fibril/tubes in [25]. These anodisks usually have uniform pore size (pore diameters). TIP FULL NAME is used as the precursor to make titania nano tubes/rods. First, TIP is dissolved in ethanol to produce a TI solution. Then, in a separate beaker, a solution of ethanol (EtOH), water, and acetylacetone (ACAC) is prepared by mixing them using a magnetic stirrer. After thorough mixing, the EtOH/ACAC/water solution is added in small quantities (usually by syringe pump set-up) to the TI solution to form titania sol. The molar ratios of various reactants are chosen as given in Table 5.1. The molar ratio of TI: ACAC: H_2O: EtOH determines the wall thickness, the diameter, and the length of the nano tubes/fibrils and hence it is crucial. The anodic alumina disks are dipped in the sol for about 10 min and then dried in room temperature for 24 h.

This experiment deploys the use of 200–250 nm diameter anodisks (Whatman anodiscs—Fisher). After drying, the anodisks are heated to 400°C for 24 h. After cooling the disks, the surface films are removed by gentle polishing with sand paper. The disks are now immersed in the NaOH solution of 20 wt%; this dissolves the alumina disk and exposes the titania nano tubes/rods. The nano tubes and fibrils could then be filtered out and secured for characterization [25]. Table 5.1 shows the particle diameter as a function of the alumina wall thickness, the ratio of reactants, and the corresponding dipping time.

5.2.3   Overview of Other Synthesis Methods
5.2.3 A)   Sol-gel synthesis by ultrasound-irradiation of TiO_2

This technique involves the synthesis of nanosized TiO_2 particles via ultrasonic irradiation [15]. This process is a combination of sol gel synthesis + hydrolysis of titanium isopropoxide and ultrasonication, done by adding to pure water, titanium isopropoxide (TIP) in drops and stirring vigorously. Later, the solution is centrifuged for 6 h at 3500 rpm. Then ultrasonic irradiation, in an ultrasonic clean bath (Branson, USA, 115 V, 2 kW, 38 kHz) is carried for 1 h. The sample is washed in distilled water and centrifuged for 10 min at 10 000 rpm and dried at 100°C for 24 h. After drying, the sample is calcined at 300–700°C for 3 h. Particle size varying from 5.1 to 21.6 nm with increasing size with increased temperature of calcinations is obtained. TiO_2 of 14 nm size is obtained for the ultrasound irradiated process, while the nonirradiated process yielded a particle size of 22 nm [15].

5.2.3 B) Microemulsion-based synthesis of TiO$_2$

A method of synthesis of titania NP via the micro-emulsion technique, the following has the materials required and the method in detail.

Reactants. A polyoxyethylene (20) sorbitan monolaurate, monopalmitate, monostearate, and trioleate (Tween 20, 60, and 85, respectively) with a different hydrophobic group and Brij 52 (polyoxyethylene glycol hexadecyl ether polyoxyethylene- 2-cetyl ether), Brij 56 (polyoxyethylene glycol hexadecyl ether polyoxyethylene-10-cetyl ether), Brij 58 (polyoxyethylene glycol hexadecyl ether polyoxyethylene-20-cetyl ether) with different hydrophilic groups are used in the synthesis [14].

The purpose (hyrophile-lipohphile balance) of choosing these hydrophilic/hydrophobic groups could be found elsewhere [14].

Method. This method involves the hydrolysis of titanium tetraisopropoxide (TTIP) in W/O microemulsions comprising of water, tween series surfactants of various hydrophobic groups, and cyclohexane. A reverse microemulsion solution is prepared by mixing 0.045 mol of surfactants in cyclohexane. To this solution the required amount of distilled water is added. After mixing, a water-clear appearance of the solution indicates the formation of microemulsion [14]. The hydrolysis of TTIP was carried out at 30°C in a sealed four-way flask (500 ml). The reaction is initiated by adding the TTIP solution into the reverse microemulsion amidst constant stirring for about 1 h. The titania particles precipitated. The resulting sample is then subjected to centrifugation at 10,000 rpm for 2 min. The precipitate is then washed with ethanol in a Soxhelt extractor for about 24 h to remove any organic/surfactants on the particles. The secured particles are then dried at 105°C for 12 h and later calcined for 3 h at 200–800°C. This process yields titania nanoparticles varying from 9 through 17 nm [14].

5.3
5.3.1 The Solid-Vapor Synthesis of ZnO: Horizontal Tube Furnace

The solid-vapor evaporation process involves the evaporation of a condensed or powdered material (of interest—ZnO) into its vapor phase which is later allowed to condense under desired conditions of pressure, temperature, atmosphere, etc. to form the predefined structures of the product. Generally this synthesis technique involves the use of a furnace as shown in Fig. A5.3.1, in which the aforementioned process is carried out [28]. The horizontal tube furnace comprises of a horizontal furnace, an alumina tube, a rotary pump, and a gas supply system. A view window is provisioned at the left end of the alumina tube to facilitate the monitoring of the synthesis process from the outside. The right-side end of the alumina tube is

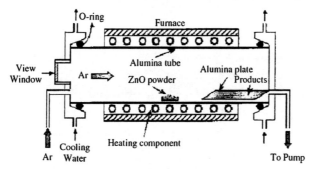

FIGURE A5.3.1: Construction of a horizontal tube furnace used for the synthesis of ZnO nanostructures by the solid-vapor method

connected to the rotary pump. Further details of the synthesis technique and the operational of the furnace could be referred elsewhere. The key point to be noted is that the parameters that dictate the fate (morphology, size, etc.) of the product are the temperature, the pressure, the atmosphere, the substrate, time of evaporation, and the flux of gas [28].

5.3.2   Wurtzite Structure of ZnO

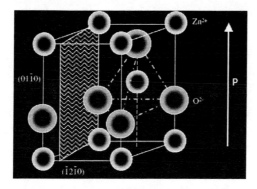

FIGURE A5.3.2: The wurtzite structure model of ZnO. The tetrahedral coordination of Zn–O is shown

REFERENCES

[1]   M. Brust, et al., "Synthesis and reactions of functionalized gold nanoparticles," *J. Chem. Soc., Chem. Commun.*, (16), pp. 1655–1656, 1995, DOI: 10.1039/C39950001655.

[2]   M. Brust, et al., "Synthesis of thiol-derivatized gold nanoparticles in a two-phase liquid-liquid system," *J. Chem. Soc., Chem. Commun.*, (7), pp. 801–2, 1994.

[3]   I. Doron-Mor, et al., "Ultrathin gold island films on silanized glass," Morphology and optical properties. *Chem. Mater.*, **16**(18), pp. 3476–3483, 2004.

[4]   K. C. Grabar, et al., "Nanoscale characterization of gold colloid monolayers: a comparison of four techniques," *Anal. Chem.*, **69**(3), pp. 471–477, 1997.

[5]   N. R. Jana, L. Gearheart, and C. J. Murphy, "Wet chemical synthesis of high aspect ratio cylindrical gold nanorods," *J. Phys. Chem. B*, **105**(19), pp. 4065–4067, 2001.

[6]   B. R. Martin, et al., "Orthogonal self-assembly on colloidal gold-platinum nanorods," *Adv. Mater.*, **11**(12), pp. 1021–1025, 1999.

[7]   D. M. Stefanescu, et al., "Synthesis and characterization of phosphido-monolayer-protected gold nanoclusters," *Langmuir*, **20**(24), pp. 10379–10381, 2004.

[8]   V. Subramanian, E. E. Wolf, and P. V. Kamat, "Catalysis with TiO2/gold nanocomposites," Effect of metal particle size on the Fermi level equilibration. *J. Am. Chem. Soc.*, **126**(15), pp. 4943–4950, 2004.

[9]   Y. Tan, et al., "Preparation of gold, platinum, palladium and silver nanoparticles by the reduction of their salts with a weak reductant-potassium bitartrate," *J. Mater. Chem.*, **13**(5), pp. 1069–1075, 2003.

[10] C. B. Almquist, and P. Biswas, "Role of synthesis method and particle size of nanostructured TiO2 on its photoactivity," *J. Catal.*, **212**(2), pp. 145–156, 2002.

[11] Z. Ding, G. Q. Lu, and P. F. Greenfield, "A kinetic study on photocatalytic oxidation of phenol in water by silica-dispersed titania nanoparticles," *J. Coll. Interface Sci.*, **232**(1), pp. 1–9, 2000.

[12] S.-S. Hong, et al., "Synthesis of nanosized TiO2/SiO2 particles in the microemulsion and their photocatalytic activity on the decomposition of p-nitrophenol," *Catal. Today*, **87**(1–4), pp. 99–105, 2003.

[13] A. A. Ismail, "Synthesis and characterization of Y2O3/Fe2O3/TiO2 nanoparticles by sol-gel method," *Appl. Catal., B, Environ.*, **58**(1–2), pp. 115–121, 2005.

[14] M. S. Lee, et al., "Synthesis of TiO2 particles by reverse microemulsion method using nonionic surfactants with different hydrophilic and hydrophobic group and their photocatalytic activity," *Catal. Today*, **101**(3–4), pp. 283–290, 2005.

[15] C. W. Oh, et al., "Synthesis of nanosized TiO2 particles via ultrasonic irradiation and their photocatalytic activity," *Reaction Kinetics Catal. Lett.*, **85**(2), pp. 261–268, 2005.

[16] J. Shim, et al., "Transdermal delivery of mixnoxidil with block copolymer nanoparticles," *J. Control. Rel.*, **97**(3), pp. 477–84, 2004.

[17] N. Uekawa, et al., "Low temperature synthesis and characterization of porous anatase TiO2 nanoparticles," *J. Coll. Interface Sci.*, **250**(2), pp. 285–290, 2002.

[18] S. H. Bossmann, et al., "Ru(bpy)32+/TiO2-codoped zeolites: synthesis, characterization, and the role of TiO2 in electron transfer photocatalysis," *J. Phys. Chem. B*, **105**(23), pp. 5374–5382, 2001.

[19] T. Tatsuma, et al., "Energy storage of TiO2-WO3 photocatalysis systems in the gas phase," *Langmuir*, **18**(21), pp. 7777–7779, 2002.

[20] C.-S. Kim, et al., "Synthesis of nanocrystalline TiO2 in toluene by a solvothermal route," *J. Cryst. Growth*, **254**(3–4), pp. 405–410, 2003.

[21] J. C. Hulteen and C. R. Martin, "A general template-based method for the preparation of nanomaterials," *J. Mater. Chem.*, **7**(7), pp. 1075–1087, 1997.

[22] B. B. Lakshmi, P. K. Dorhout, and C. R. Martin, "Sol-gel template synthesis of semiconductor nanostructures," *Chem. Mater.*, **9**(3), pp. 857–862, 1997.

[23] B. B. Lakshmi and C. R. Martin, "Sol-gel template synthesis of semiconductor nanostructures," *Proceedings—Electrochemical Society*, vol. 97–11(Quantum Confinement: Nanoscale Materials, Devices, and Systems), pp. 47–55, 1997.

[24] B. B. Lakshmi, C. J. Patrissi, and C.R. Martin, "Sol-gel template synthesis of semiconductor oxide micro- and nanostructures," *Chem. Mater.*, **9**(11), pp. 2544–2550, 1997.

[25] M. Zhang, Y. Bando, and K. Wada, "Sol-gel template preparation of TiO2 nanotubes and nanorods," *J. Mater. Sci. Lett.*, **20**(2), pp. 167–170, 2001.

[26] Y. Nakanishi and T. Imae, "Synthesis of dendrimer-protected TiO2 nanoparticles and photodegradation of organic molecules in an aqueous nanoparticle suspension," *J. Coll. Interface Sci.*, **285**(1), pp. 158–162, 2005.

[27] Y. Bessekhouad, D. Robert, and J. V. Weber, "Synthesis of photocatalytic TiO2 nanoparticles: optimization of the preparation conditions," *J. Photochem. Photobiol., A: Chem.*, **157**(1), pp. 47–53, 2003.

[28] Z. L. Wang, "Zinc oxide nanostructures: growth, properties and applications," *J. Phys.: Condens. Matter*, **16**(25), p. R829, 2004.

[29] C. Ye, et al., "Zinc oxide nanostructures: morphology derivation and evolution," *J. Phys. Chem. B*, **109**(42), pp. 19758–19765, 2005.

[30] P. X. Gao, Y. Ding, and Z. L. Wang, "Crystallographic orientation-aligned ZnO nanorods grown by a tin catalyst," *Nano Lett.*, **3**(9), pp. 1315–1320, 2003.

[31] J. L. H. Chik, S. G. Cloutier, N. Kouklin, and J. M. Xu, "Periodic array of uniform ZnO nanorods by second-order self-assembly," *Appl. Phys. Lett.*, **84**(17), pp. 3376–78, 2004.

[32] Z. L. Wang, "Functional oxide nanobelts: materials, properties and potential applications in nanosystems and biotechnology," *Ann. Rev. Phys. Chem.*, **55**(1), pp. 159–196, 2004.

[33] Z. W. Pan, Z. R. Dai, and Z. L. Wang, "Nanobelts of semiconducting oxides," *Science*, **291**(5510), pp. 1947–1949, 2001.

[34] X. D. Wang, Y. D., C. J. Summers and Z. L. Wang, "Large-scale synthesis of six-nanometer-wide ZnO nanobelts," *J. Phys. Chem. B*, **108**, pp. 8773–8777, 2004.

[35] A. S. Barnard, Y. Xiao, and Z. Cai, "Modelling the shape and orientation of ZnO nanobelts," *Chem. Phys. Lett.*, **419**(4–6), p. 313, 2006.

[36] Z. L. Wang, X. Y. Kong, and J. M. Zuo, "Induced growth of asymmetric nanocantilever arrays on polar surfaces," *Phys. Rev. Lett.*, **91**(18), p. 185502, 2003.

[37] S. Yu, et al., "Precursor induced synthesis of hierarchical nanostructured ZnO," *Nanotechnology*, **17**(14), p. 3607, 2006.

[38] X. S. Yaohua Zhang1, J. Z. Haihua Liu2, and a. L. Y. Xingguo Li1, 4, "Symmetric and asymmetric growth of ZnO hierarchical nanostructures: nanocombs and their optical properties," *Nanotechnology*, **17**, pp. 1916–21, 2006.

[39] S. Hashimoto and A. Yamaguchi, "Growth morphology and mechanism of a hollow ZnO polycrystal," *J. Am. Ceram. Soc.*, **79**(4), pp. 1121–1123, 1996.

[40] D. Moore, et al., "Wurtzite ZnS nanosaws produced by polar surfaces," *Chem. Phys. Lett.*, **385**(1–2), p. 8, 2004.

[41] P. X. G. Chang Shi Lao, Ru Sen Yang, Yue Zhang, and Y. D. a. Z. L. Wang, "Formation of double-side teethed nanocombs of ZnO and self-catalysis of Zn-terminated polar surface," *Chem. Phys. Lett.*, **417**, pp. 359–363, 2005.

[42] X. Y. Kong and Z. L. Wang, "Spontaneous polarization-induced nanohelixes, nanosprings, and nanorings of piezoelectric nanobelts," *Nano Lett.*, **3**(12), pp. 1625–1631, 2003.

[43] H. Soon-Ku, et al. "Control of ZnO film polarity," Journal of Vacuum Science & Technology B: Microelectronics and Nanometer Structures. Vol. **20**(4), pp. 1656–1663, 2002.

[44] K. Xiang Yang and W. Zhong Lin, "Polar-surface dominated ZnO nanobelts and the electrostatic energy induced nanohelixes, nanosprings, and nanospirals," *Appl. Phys. Lett.*, **84**(6), pp. 975–977, 2004.

[45] X. Y. Kong, et al., "Single-crystal nanorings formed by epitaxial self-coiling of polar nanobelts," *Science*, **303**(5662), pp. 1348–1351, 2004.

[46] H. Dai, et al., "Nanotubes as nanoprobes in scanning probe microscopy," *Nature*, **384**(6605), p. 147, 1996.

[47] L. H. William and L. W. Zhong, "Nanobelts as nanocantilevers," *Appl. Phys. Lett.*, **82**(17), pp. 2886–2888, 2003.

[48] M. H. Zhao, Z. L. Wang, and S. X. Mao, "Piezoelectric characterization of individual zinc oxide nanobelt probed by piezoresponse force microscope," *Nano Lett.*, **4**(4), pp. 587–590, 2004.

[49] C. S. Rout, et al., "Hydrogen and ethanol sensors based on ZnO nanorods, nanowires and nanotubes," *Chem. Phys. Lett.*, **418**(4–6), p. 586, 2006.

CHAPTER 6

Is Bionanotechnology a Panacea?

AN INSIGHT INTO NANO TOXICOLOGY

Introduction. The use of bionanotechnology in Medicine and Health Care depends on design, synthesis, modification, and detection of "smart" nano-entities that actively or passively contribute to diagnosis and therapy [1, 2]. It is necessary to establish the long-term safety of the use of nanoparticles in humans, not only during therapy but also during manufacturing or any other means of unintended exposure [3]. This chapter addresses toxicological aspects of bionanotechnology related to the presence of nanosize entities in the human body and the consequences of their transport and interaction with human tissues and organs. Issues of economic, social, and ethical concern in bionanotechnology applications are also briefly discussed. This is an area of intense current activity and focus by the international community [4–8].

6.1   BACKGROUND

The medical and heath care industry harvests the unique properties of nanomaterials by employing nano-manufacturing techniques and processes to yield nano entities for specific applications. Bionanotechnology is a new technology that is in the phase of drastic growth and development [1, 2]. During this early growth phase, issues concerning the possible toxic long-term impact of nanoparticles (NPs) during use, manufacture, disposal, and environmental exposure have not yet been fully explored [9, 10]. The following section discusses health, environmental, and safety aspects of nanotechnology applications in biology and medicine and charts the necessary steps to address and answer some of these questions.

6.2   PRIMARY CONCERNS

The key features of nanoparticles are their small size, their higher surface area, the special optical properties based on semiconducting materials, and possibly the specialty-coating surface coating [1, 11, 12]. These same features, however, enhance their activity when they enter the human body, and raise questions regarding systemic effects and long-term toxicity [11, 13]. A recurring theme is the ability of nanoparticles to cross cell membranes [14] and due to their high surface reactivity cause human and environmental toxicity [15]? If this tissue and cell permeability is indeed happening, are there limits of safe exposure? Do the particles clear the body after a certain time without adverse effects, or is there a long-term exposure issue? How can we define the limits of safe use of nanoparticles? The same issues faced by bionanotechnology today have already been faced by today's mature materials such as plastics [16]. Plastics, once known to be the materials of the future, have undergone increased scrutiny and their use and manufacture evolved in ways to minimize environmental impact. No one can underestimate the impact of NPs as they can easily be transported and remain undetected propagating through the food chain and infiltrating into organisms at any level or hierarchy.

The very size of nanoparticles, lying in the nm range, is less than or equal to cellular system components and associated sub-units like proteins [17]. It seems therefore plausible that NPs could intrude and defeat host defenses [14, 17, 18]. The fact that NPs could even cross the blood brain barrier [19–22], as mentioned in *Chapter 2* of drug delivery, introduces the need for long-term studies of possible long-term health effects.

6.3   ASSESSING POTENTIAL RISKS

Government and research agencies have implemented laws and regulations on the use of airborn particles or other known harmful materials that could cause potential threat to human health, upon exposure in manufacturing, synthesis, and disposal, when the toxic effects are demonstrated and quantified with specific exposure levels. Similar studies will have to be conducted with nanoparticles to assess their risk and limits of safe usage [9].

In order to assess the impact of nanoparticles on human health and the environment we would need to:

- Identify potential threats and hazard.
- Determine the probability of exposure to the hazard.
- Perform life cycle analysis of the NPs.
- Control the nano-materials released in air water or through the food chain.
- Establish limits of safe usage.
- Devise methods and implement practices to control possible hazards.

Possible adverse effects of nanoparticle exposure can occur if there is systemic exposure and nanoparticles can enter the human body via inhalation, ingestion, transdermal penetration, or intended delivery in the blood stream. The following conditions must be met therefore:

- The NP comes in contact with the body
- The minimum dose to evoke body reactions is delivered into the body
- The particles reach its target

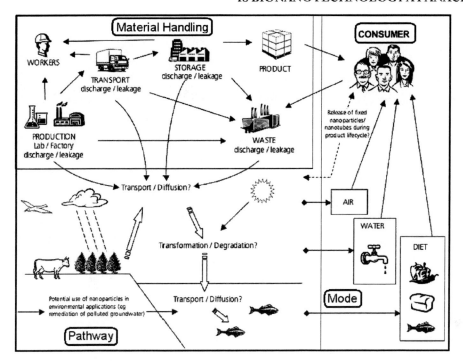

FIGURE 6.1: Sources, pathway, and routes of invasion of NPs into the human body

The above conditions could be facilitated through the following pathways –

- By direct inhalation
- By ingestion of the NP by the human being
- Contact—via skin
- Via medication—drugs, medicines, injections, and other routes
- Infected members of food chain—bacteria (lower level members)

It is quite evident from the disputes and discussions that nanotechnology needs a lot of further research on areas of toxicology studies, exposure studies, health hazard impacts, risk evaluation, and management to find an optimal solution that will serve human health taking advantage of the breakthrough potential of bionanotechnology [10, 23, 24].

Fig. 6.1 shows the various sources, pathways, and modes (routes) through which NPs of a particular material may reach the human body [4, 25]. There are several sources of delivering nanoparticles to the environment and then NPs may intrude into the integral units of the ecosystem.

6.3.1   Inhalation

Inhalation of NPs of various materials leads to pulmonary diseases [17, 26–35]. NPs have a high probability to reach the lungs due to their small size [23, 36]. They easily escape the body's immune response (macrophages) as they may be too small to evoke a foreign body response. At the same time the risk associated with entering and interfering with the cellular machinery is high. Currently, commercial scale production of NPs includes zinc oxide, titania, iron oxide, gold nanoparticles, quantum dots, and carbon nano tubes, and the list is expanding at a fast rate. Manufacturing causes direct exposure of NPs to the workers in the environment and there is a high probability of such particles entering the lungs in larger numbers [37], the case is same with exposures occurring during research activities [4]. Opportunities to improve synthesis processes of nanoparticles to a closed loop system minimizing exposure and waste must be given priority.

It is safer to think of handling nano-materials as hazardous/toxic entity and provide professionals who handle them with adequate protection hygiene, respiratory protection, protection against skin/contact etc [4]. It is also important to educate the professionals on the hazardous nature of the NPs and train them to handle accidents, emissions, spills.

Synthetic NP may contain residual catalysts used in their synthesis or in the preparation of surface coatings surrounding them. For instance, CNT synthesis uses iron or other metals as catalysts and as a result minute traces of iron are maintained within these tubes [38]. The presence of iron/other metals could be associated with the CNT ability to produce free radicals and provoke pro-inflammatory responses [38]. A dosage of 60–240 µg of single wall CNTs is considered to be a high dose for epithelial exposure. Manufacturing plants of CNTs must be strictly viewed as hazardous environment and implement safety measures. CNT, especially the single wall carbon nano tubes (SWCNT) are known to be quite harmful to humans [39].

6.3.2   Contact/Dermal Delivery

The dermal route is another pathway though which NPs may enter the human body, either from accidental exposure during manufacturing or from unintended use of a skin formulation (cosmetic or pharmaceutical) that contains "inert" nanoparticles. Popular NPs used in dermal formulations include titania and zinc oxide sun locks, iron oxide based lipsticks, face creams [4]. While titania is a scientifically proven safer material [40, 41], it does not cross the epidermis too and is quite safe to be used in any size with/without surface coatings [4, 40]. However, the case is not the same with zinc oxide nanoparticles. The recent concerns raised on the European counterpart of FDA, the Scientific Committee on Cosmetic and Non-Food Products (SCC-NFP), on inadequate disclosure of toxic studies of nanoparticle contained dermal formulations [42] must serve as an example of pro-active studies that need to be undertaken [43]. FDA had earlier approved zinc oxide to be used as a sun screen without size restrictions [44]; however it is notable that ZnO NPs of size lesser than 200 nm (micro-fine) exhibit photo-toxic effects on mammalian cells *in vitro* [43] and is a matter of raising concern [4]. Further studies are required to ascertain the *in vivo* characteristics of nano-size zinc oxide.

6.3.3   Other Routes of Contact

Nanoparticles may simultaneously enter the body through multiple routes of entry and one wonders if this creates increased risks of exposure of NPs to the body. The shape, size, surface charge, and deformability of the particle will play a key role on its interaction with the body and determine exposure risks [12]. To answer the above questions, significant research needs to be done in these areas with close involvement of scientists, nanotech experts, and toxicologists to examine every possible situation of threat.

6.3.4   Environmental Impacts of NPs and the Food Chain

Let us consider a food-chain as shown in Fig. 6.2, which shows man at the top of the food-chain hierarchy. The food chain represented here has many integral members such as the aquatic life, air, soil, etc. (not shown) in which the living beings of various levels thrive. There is great possibility of NPs polluting the food-chain and the ecosystem as well.

A pilot study suggests the possible harmful impacts of C_{60} on the brains of the fish to which they were exposed [45]. The study-results indicate higher oxidation of fats in the brain

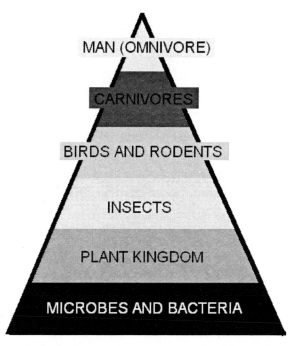

FIGURE 6.2: Schematic of a food-chain with man at the topmost hierarchy

of the fish, though the results were at lower concentration, while it happens that the study indicates a possible long-term harmful effects of NPs on aquatic life [45, 46]. Further, there are several thousand microbial organisms, sea weeds, plants, and other aquatic members which are a part of the food-chain; thus pollution of the environment takes less time to affect humans.

Nanoparticles may pollute the environment through their persistence, bioaccumulation, and toxicity. This is why "inert" nanoparticles although non-toxic could cause environmental damage due to their persistence or bioaccumulation potential.

Apart from the toxic studies carried out in humans and animals care must be taken to other aspects of NPs pollution. For instance, the physical and chemical properties of NPs subjected to various environmental conditions, their ability to react with the environment, their stability, their active life-time, their abilities to agglomerate [6], etc.

Soil and water pollution by NPs is a significant potential threat to the environment and human health, because it will affect vegetables, fruits, plants, etc. Fertilizers meant to nourish the soil, which contain NPs, may also cause adverse effects. For instance, the ground water pollution by iron nanoparticles is worth notable [47]. Thus, soil studies and materials employed as fertilizers and in remediation need to be studied for interactions with the environment as well as for long-term toxic effects. The longer we allow nanoparticles to accumulate unnoticed in the environment, the faster their levels may reach toxic potential [4]. For instance, iron nanoparticles could travel up to 20 m in the ground water-table, while being active for 4–8 weeks [47], thus posing a potential threat to invade the members of a food chain at any given hierarchy.

6.3.5 Explosion Hazards

Dust explosions caused by adequate nano-powder discharges in air are a potential threat that also needs to be addressed. Manufacturing plants of nano-powders, nano-tubes, nano-materials, plastics, metallic powders, organic chemicals, sawdust, etc. are potential places where dust explosion may occur [48]. The data available for macro-scale particles and their dust explosion risk cannot be simply extrapolated to nano-size particles. Further, the severity of an explosion and its relation to particle size is speculative and needs to be ascertained with adequate research [48]. However, high heat treatment of nano/particles needs to be avoided or performed in constant cooling or a liquid medium (colloidal preparations). For example, carbon-black processing is safer if one avoids rotary driers where high heat is generated [4, 48].

6.4 LESSONS FROM THE PAST

A summary of the path followed to assess adverse effects of other new materials that resemble nanoparticles could serve as a roadmap to the necessary steps for the safe use of nanoparticles. *Quartz, for example is* a mineral of silicon di-oxide, found in abundance on the earth's surface.

Often mining workers are exposed to high quantities of minute particles of quartz [49]. Lung fibrosis leading to fatal conditions is a result of high concentration exposure to quartz. It has become now known through rigorous research efforts that the surface of quartz particles is highly reactive oxidizing cell membranes and causing inflammation, cell death, fibrosis, and tumors [50–52]. *Asbestos belongs to a family* of fibrous metamorphic minerals of the hydrous magnesium silicate variety. It is naturally available in various structures and is being used for applications such as heat-resistant sheets, gaskets, brake shoes, etc. In 1918, a US insurance company brought to light the labor deaths caused in asbestos industries [53, 54]. An article titled "Mortality from respiratory diseases in dusty (inorganic) trades," further described the role of asbestos in premature death of workers [55]. Asbestos fibers less than 3 μm (aspect ratio 3) can easily reach the lungs. After reaching the lungs, they cause foreign body response and initiate the recruiting of macrophages, triggering a chain of foreign body processes ending up in scarring or lung cancer [56, 57]. Other asbestos-related diseases include asbestosis, mesothelioma (cancer), cancer of the larynx, etc [58]. *Air pollution* and its impact on human health and the environment is a classical example that needs to be studied in depth to understand the critical aspects of small-sized particles and their interactions with living matter. Particulate entities of the air pollution are said to cause not only inflammations [4, 52], lung diseases [27, 50, 59], but also cardiovascular diseases [60–63], it even extends to reach the brain as observed in the case of urban dogs [64]. One of the best known sources contributing to air pollution is combustion, where burning of a material in the presence of oxygen gives off a lot of heat and gaseous combustion byproducts. These gases, upon condensation yield nanoparticles ranging from 10 nm to 100 nm [4]. Deaths due to air pollution have been associated with the nanoparticles present in the pollution streams. The infamous London smog of 1952 killed almost 4000+ people, drawing the attention of the international community.

Extending the knowledge gained from studies of quartz, asbestos, and air pollution to the nano-entities of value in biomedical applications we can summarize the key variables that may affect nanoparticle toxicity:

1. The surface activity of a material [12, 16, 46, 57, 65] (native or surface coated [35])
2. The total surface area of the NP exposed to the organ/tissues [4, 23, 46].
3. The dose of the NP delivered [4, 23, 38, 66].
4. The solubility of the NPs [4, 35] (it would be inversely proportional to toxicity and damage)
5. Length and diameter of the NPs, especially aspect ratio [26, 57].
6. Size (nano vs. micro) and deformability that allows entrance into the body [4, 36, 67]
7. Ability to produce free radicals [38, 45, 46].

6.5 CONCLUSION

Comprehensive data and studies on long-term effects of NPs on humans and the environment need to be completed in order to create a rational basis for the open-minded acceptance of bionanotechnology application. If adverse effects are discovered, toxic exposure levels must be established and plans developed to address overexposure or release scenarios. To address toxicological aspects as well as ethical issues, scientists from industry and academia on nanotechnology, biomedical applications and medicine, business leaders, environmental experts, and law makers must work in highly inter-disciplinary research teams to study, quantify, and estimate the NPs safety. The global aspects of nanoparticle burden on the environment must also be addressed.

REFERENCES

[1] W. C. W. Chan, "Bionanotechnology Progress and Advances," *Biol. Blood Marrow Transplant.*, vol. **12**, pp. 87–91, 2006.

[2] O. V. Salata, "Application of nanoparticles in biology and medicine," *J. Nanobiotechnol.*, vol. **2**, p. 3, 2004.

[3] 3i, Nanotechnology—size matters building a successful nanotechnology company, *E.I.U.a.t.I.o. Nanotechnology.*, 2002.

[4] T. R. S.-B. Govt., The Royal Society Report—'Nanoscience and nanotechnologies: opportunities and uncertainties'. *Nanosci. Nanotechnol.*, pp. 1–111, 2004.

[5] R. J. a. A. G. Stephen Wood, *Economic and Social Research Council (ESRC): Social and Economic Challenges of Nanotechnology.* 2005 [cited; Available from: http://www.esrcsocietytoday.ac.uk/ESRCInfoCentre/about/CI/CP/research%5Fpublications/.

[6] J. S. M. Tsuji, D. Howard Andrew, C. James Paul, T. Lam John, Warheit Chiuwing, B. Santamaria David, B. Annette, "Research strategies for safety evaluation of nanomaterials, part IV: risk assessment of nanoparticles," *Toxicol. Sci.*, vol. **89**(1), pp. 42–50, 2006.

[7] C. Phoenix, and E. Drexler, "Safe exponential manufacturing," *Nanotechnology*, vol. **15**(8), p. 869, 2004.

[8] M. C Roco, "The US National Nanotechnology Initiative after 3 years (2001–2003)," *J. Nanopart. Res.*, vol. **6**(1), pp. 1–10, 2004.

[9] A. A. Shvedova, et al., "Unusual inflammatory and fibrogenic pulmonary responses to single-walled carbon nanotubes in mice," *Am. J. Physiol. Lung Cell Mol. Physiol.*, vol. **289**(5), pp. L698–708, 2005.

[10] M. D. Mehta, From biotechnology to nanotechnology: what can we learn from earlier technologies? *Bull. Sci. Technol. Soc.*, vol. **24**(1), pp. 34–39, 2004.

[11] V. E. Kagan, H. Bayir, and A. A. Shvedova, Nanomedicine and nanotoxicology: two sides of the same coin. Nanomed.: *Nanotechnol., Biol. Med.*, vol. **1**(4), p. 313, 2005.

[12] M. Geiser, S. Schurch, and P. Gehr, "Influence of surface chemistry and topography of particles on their immersion into the lung's surface-lining layer," *J. Appl. Physiol.*, vol. **94**, pp. 1793–1801, 2003.

[13] H. M. Kipen, and D. L. Laskin, Smaller is not always better: nanotechnology yields nanotoxicology. *Am. J. Physiol. Lung Cell. Mol. Physiol.*, vol. **289**(5), pp. L696–697, 2005.

[14] L. C. Renwick, K. Donaldson, and A. Clouter, "Impairment of alveolar macrophage phagocytosis by ultrafine particles," *Toxicol. Appl. Pharmacol.*, vol. **172**(2), p. 119, 2001.

[15] R. F. Service, "Nanomaterials show signs of toxicity," *Science*, vol. **300**, p. 243, 2003.

[16] S. R. BMRB, *Nanotechnology: Views of the General Public [Quantitative and qualitative research carried out as part of the Nanotechnology study]*, pp. 1–68, 2004.

[17] E. Bermudez, et al., "Pulmonary responses of mice, rats, and hamsters to subchronic inhalation of ultrafine titanium dioxide particles," *Toxicol. Sci.*, vol. **77**(2), pp. 347–357, 2004.

[18] M. C. Lomer, R. P. Thompson, and J. J. Powell, Fine and ultrafine particles of the diet: influence on the mucosal immune response and association with Crohn's disease. *Proc. Nutr. Soc.*, vol. **61**, pp. 123–130, 2002.

[19] R. N. Alyaudtin, et al., "Interaction of poly(butylcyanoacrylate) nanoparticles with the blood-brain barrier in vivo and in vitro," *J Drug Target*, vol. **9**, pp. 209–221, 2001.

[20] U. Schroeder, et al., "Nanoparticle technology for delivery of drugs across the blood-brain barrier," *J. Pharm. Sci.*, vol. **87**, pp. 1305–1307, 1998.

[21] J. Kreuter, "Nanoparticulate systems for brain delivery of drugs," *Adv. Drug Deliv. Rev.*, vol. **47**, pp. 65–81, 2001.

[22] G. Oberdörster, et al., "Translocation of inhaled ultrafine particles to the brain," *Inhal. Toxicol.*, vol. **16**, pp. 437–445, 2004.

[23] P. Hoet, I. Bruske-Hohlfeld, and O. Salata, "Nanoparticles—known and unknown health risks," *J. Nanobiotechnol.*, vol. **2**(1), p. 12, 2004.

[24] P. S. Anto'n, R. Silberglitt, and S. James, "The Globaltechnology Revolution: Bio/Nano/Materials Trends and Their Synergies with Information Technology by 2015," RAND: National Defense Research Institute, Sanata Monica, CA. pp. 1–87, 2001.

[25] NIRE. *Evaluation Technologies for Environmental Effects and Ecotechnology: Impacts on our surroundings*. [cited 2006 10/08/2006]; Image]. Available from: http://www.nire.go.jp/eco_tec_e/hyouka_e.htm.

[26] S. H. Moolgavkar, R. C. Brown, and J. Turim, "Biopersistence, fiber length, and cancer risk assessment for inhaled fibers," *Inhal Toxicol*, vol. **13**, pp. 755–772, 2001.

[27] M. Lippmann, Effects of fiber characteristics on lung deposition, retention, and disease. Environ. *Health Perspect.*, vol. **88**, pp. 311–317, 1990.

[28] G. Oberdorster, "Pulmonary effects of inhaled ultrafine particles," *Int. Arch. Occup. Environ. Health*, vol. **74**, pp. 1–8, 2001.

[29] G. Oberdorster, "Toxicokinetics and effects of fibrous and nonfibrous particles," *Inhal. Toxicol.*, vol. **14**, pp. 29–56, 2002.

[30] D. B. Warheit, et al., "Potential pulmonary effects of man-made organic fiber (MMOF) dusts," *Crit. Rev. Toxicol.*, vol. **31**, pp. 697–736, 2001.

[31] D. B. Warheit, et al., "Comparative pulmonary toxicity assessment of single wall carbon nanotubes in rats," *Toxicol. Sci.*, vol. **77**, pp. 117–125, 2003.

[32] U. Heinrich, et al., "Pulmonary function changes in rats after chronic and subchronic inhalation exposure to various particulate matter," *Exp. Pathol.*, vol. **37**, pp. 248–252, 1989.

[33] K. P. Lee, et al., "Inhalation toxicity study on rats exposed to titanium tetrachloride atmospheric hydrolysis products for two years," *Toxicol. Appl. Pharmacol.*, vol. **83**, pp. 30–45, 1986.

[34] G. Oberdorster, et al., "Extrapulmonary translocation of ultrafine carbon particle following whole-body inhalation exposure of rats," *J. Toxicol. Environ. Health A*, vol. **65**, pp. 1531–1543, 2002.

[35] P. J. A. Borm, and W. Kreyling, Toxicological hazards of inhaled nanoparticles – potential implications for drug delivery. *J. Nanosci. Nanotechnol.*, vol. **4**, pp. 1–11, 2004.

[36] G. Oberdorster, J. Ferin, and B. E. Lehnert, "Correlation between particle size, in vivo particle persistence, and lung injury," *Environ. Health Perspect.*, vol. **102**, pp. 173–179, 1994.

[37] G. Oberdorster, Lung particle overload: implications for occupational exposures to particles. *Regul. Toxicol. Pharmacol.*, **21**, pp. 123–135, 1995.

[38] A. A. Shvedova, et al., Exposure to carbon nanotube material: assessment of nanotube cytotoxicity usung human keratinocyte cells. *J. Toxicol. Environ. Health Part A*, vol. **66**(20), pp. 1909–1926, 2003.

[39] D. B. Warheit, et al., "Comparative pulmonary toxicity assessment of single-wall carbon nanotubes in rats," *Toxicol. Sci.*, vol. **77**(1), pp. 117–125, 2004.

[40] SCCNFP, Opinion of the scientific committee on cosmetic products and non-food products intended for consumers on titanium dioxide (Colipa no S75), pp. 1–38, 2000.

[41] Bennat and G. Muller, "Skin penetration and stabilization of formulations containing microfine titanium dioxide as physical UV filter," *Int. J. Cosmetic Sci.*, vol. **22**(4), pp. 271–283, 2000.

[42] SCCNFP, The SCCNFPs notes of guidance for the testing of cosmetic ingredients and their safety evaluation, pp. 1–114, 2000.

[43] SCCNFP, The scientific committee on cosmetic products and non-food products (sccnfp) intended for consumers opinion concerning zinc oxide (COLIPA no S 76). pp. 1–31, 2003.

[44] H. Food and Drug Administration, "Rules and regulations: sunscreen drug products for over-the-counter human use," *Final Monograph*, D.O.H.A.H. SERVICES, pp. 27666–27693, 1999.

[45] E. Oberdörster, "Manufactured nanomaterials (fullerenes, C60) induce oxidative stress in the brain of juvenile largemouth bass," *Environ. Health Perspect.*, vol. **12**(10), pp. 1058–1062, 2004.

[46] M. N. Moore, Do nanoparticles present ecotoxicological risks for the health of the aquatic environment? *Environ. Int.*; **32**(8), pp. 967–76, 2006.

[47] W. -x. Zhang, "Nanoscale iron particles for environmental remediation: an overview," *J. Nanopart. Res.*, vol. **5**(3–4), pp. 323–332, 2003.

[48] D. K. Pritchard, "Literature review—explosion hazards associated with nanopowders," *Health and Safety Laboratory*, pp. 1–22, 2004.

[49] International Labour, O., Safety in the use of mineral and synthetic fibres; working document and report of the meeting of experts on safety in the use of mineral and synthetic fibres, Geneva, 17–25 April 1989. *Occup. Safety Health Ser.*, vol. **64**, pp. 1–94, 1990.

[50] A. Seaton, et al., "Pneumoconiosis of shale miners," Thorax, vol. **36**(6), pp. 412–418, 1981.

[51] R. F. Service, "Nanotoxicology: nanotechnology grows up," *Science*, vol. **304**(5678), pp. 1732–1734, 2004.

[52] V. Vallyathan, "Generation of oxygen radicals by minerals and its correlation to cytotoxicity," *Environ. Health Perspect.*, vol. **102**(Suppl. 10), pp. 111–115, 1994.

[53] Unknown, Midwest Asbestos Company—Arizona 1915, in *Scripophily*.

[54] P. Wong, *Parliamentry Address—New South Wales (NSW) Legislative Council Hansard: Asbestos.* Parliament of New South Wales. p. 10492 2004.

[55] Hale, Julius, and Kershaw. *Discovering Asbestos in Rockbridge County: What is Asbestos?* 2006 [cited; Available from: http://journalism.wlu.edu/indepth/Asbestos/background.htm.

[56] D. W. Berman, et al., "The sizes, shapes, and mineralogy of asbestos structures that induce lung tumors or mesothelioma in AF/HAN rats following inhalation," *Risk Anal*, vol. **15**, pp. 181–195, 1995.

[57] J. C. Wagner, et al., "A pathological and mineralogical study of asbestos-related deaths in the United Kingdom in 1977," *Ann. Occup. Hyg.*, vol. **26**(3), pp. 423–431, 1982.

[58] Hale, Julius, and Kershaw. *Discovering Asbestos in Rockbridge County: Health Hazards.* [News Article] 2006 [cited 2006 10/09/2006]; Available from: http://journalism.wlu.edu/indepth/Asbestos/Health.htm.

[59] A. Seaton, *Silicosis. In Occupational Lung Diseases,* Eds. e.M.W.K.C.S. A. 3rd edition, (Philadelphia, USA: WB Saunders), 1995.

[60] R. D. Brook, et al., Air pollution and cardiovascular disease: a statement for healthcare professionals from the Expert Panel on Population and Prevention Science of the American Heart Association. *Circulation*, vol. **109**(21), pp. 2655–2671, 2004.

[61] D. Liao, et al., Daily variation of particulate air pollution and poor cardiac autonomic control in the elderly. *Environ. Health Perspect.*, vol. **107**, pp. 521–525, 1999.

[62] A. Peters, et al., "Increased particulate air pollution and the triggering of myocardial infarction," *Circulation*, vol. **103**, pp. 2810–2815, 2001.

[63] A. Peters, et al., "Air pollution and incidence of cardiac arrhythmia," *Epidemiology*, vol. **11**, pp. 11–17, 2000.

[64] L. Calderón-Garcidueñas, et al., "DNA damage and in nasal and brain tissue of canines exposed to air pollutants is associated with evidence of chronic brain inflammation and neurodegeneration," *Toxicol. Pathol.*, vol. **31**, pp. 524–538, 2003.

[65] V. Labhasetwar, et al., "Arterial uptake of biodegradable nanoparticles: effect of surface modifications," *J. Pharm. Sci.*, vol. **87**, pp. 1229–1234, 1998.

[66] G. Oberdörster, "Significance of particle parameters in the evaluation of exposure – dose response relationships of inhaled particles," *Inhal. Toxicol.*, vol. **8**, pp. 73–89, 1996.

[67] M. F. Stanton, et al., "Carcinogenicity of fibrous glass: pleural response in the rat in relation to fiber dimension," *J. Natl. Cancer. Inst.*, vol. **58**, pp. 587–603, 1977.

CHAPTER 7

Roadmap to Realization of Bionanotechnology

7.1   INTRODUCTION

Having so far looked into intricate details of several aspects of bionanotechnology, we now come to the concluding notes. In this chapter, we present to you a brief summary of the previous chapters and also the futuristic aspects of bionanotech. However, the core of this chapter deals with the global race and the roadmap to the realization of translation research in bionanotechnology. The unprecedented growth and development in bionanotech forecasts annual expenditure to the tune of $1 Trillion by the year 2015 in the United States-alone, the same scenario is observed globally too. Thus, it is of supreme importance to capture the global trend proceeding with bionano research.

7.2   NANO VISION: THE FUTURISTIC GOALS OF BIONANOTECH

The typical expectation of people from a developing technology is often more than realistic limits; bionanotechnology is no exception to this. The global expectation from bionanotech to cater to various needs is increasing day by day. There are several industries, of interest to us, which find direct application in bionanotechnology and there are others that are associated with bionanotech that are striving for increased contribution from nanotechnology. A list of such industries includes:

1. Precision Engineering.   This might include a top-down approach or a bottom-up approach. But the top-down approach uses various nano-lithographic techniques in creating nanodevices for MEMS [1–3] and NEMS [1, 4, 5]. While the bottom-up approach would use synthetic means of producing nano-products by building them from their molecules. Example for bottom-up approach includes synthesis of various nano-particles such as nano-tubes [6–8], nano-rods [9, 10], nano-clusters [11], other drug-capsules, etc.

2. Optics and Imaging.   The depth of application of nanotechnology has greatly influenced optics. Imaging various cells, tissues, organs, and other biological systems has come through a great journey to attain high-magnification, more resolution, and information [12–20]. Modern imaging devices such as electron microscopy, AFM [4, 21], TEM [22–24], NSOM, confocal microscopy, etc. deal with nano-details of the specimen probed.

3. Medical. The medical field in general works toward improved implant and prosthetics with better quality, life-extension, performance, and enhanced biocompatibility. The degree of roughness and smoothness in nano-biomaterials [25–27], nano-scaffolds [28–30] are defined in nm range to yield better performance.

4. Pharmaceuticals. This is one of the most booming outcome of bionanotechnology. While it is easily evident that bionanotech has immensely contributed to the development of the pharmaceutical industries and other biotech firms, it is increasingly expected of bionanotech to play an even more significant role in these fields to fulfill the present day demands. The pharmaceutical industry is driven toward nano-vector drug delivery, targeted delivery, avoiding toxicity, controlled delivery through smart-vehicles, escaping the RES, etc. [31–44].

There is no doubt that the above-mentioned fields have benefitted from ground-breaking research in bionanotech. However, the present goals set forth by various firms in drug delivery, imaging, biosensors, precision engineering, optics, nano-electronics, medicine, etc. sometimes seem too far-fetched from realization. It is widely believed and an accepted fact that many scientists and industries are mislead by the so-called nano-hype to imagine un-realistic goals to be feasible [45]. However, it is left to the present trends and the progress to decide on the realizable goals and set the pathway for the future.

7.3   WORKING TOWARD REALIZATION: CURRENT PROGRESS

We have seen the development in bionanotech in several industries, and this is quite evident from the material presented in *Chapters 1–5*. Although there are few setbacks and concerns in bionano research like the toxic effects [46–49], the current progress made in every industry is immense. The present development has encouraged more funding opportunities and further room for development. We now focus onto three industries of utmost importance to the bionano research:

- Biotechnology
- Drug Delivery
- Bio-Imaging

Biotechnology. Biotech has been revolutionized through bionano research and development. The industry now talks of nano dimensions in every aspect. For instance, the surface function-alization [14] at nano-scales is a top-priority bionano aspect, increasingly being exploited by the biotech companies. The use of anti-body, nucleic acids, other proteins, viruses, polymers, etc. to functionalize bionano entities deployed in human diagnostic/therapeutic application is a seemingly developing work in the biotech industries. The use of surface functionalization techniques enables the design of nano-vectors, unique for chosen applications [14]. Such nano-vectors are highly site-specific and multi-target capable [50]. The diagnostic and therapeutic applications which deploy the nano-vectors can be used to treat deadly conditions and diseases such as tumors [50], cancers [50], inflammations, and even chronic medical conditions such as diabetes. Drug delivery and bio-imaging form a larger part of the bionano industry; they are two important branches of the very biotech Industry, at large. The aforementioned applications hold well for both bio-imaging as well as drug-delivery/pharmaceuticals. Targeted approach to imaging and drug-delivery is of high interest today. Also, the surface functionalization techniques enable several features in the nano-vectors for drug delivery, like escaping the RES [51], avoiding overdose and toxicity [44, 52, 53], controlled [54] and site-specific delivery [16, 55], automatic-identification of tumor sites, crossing the BBB [39], etc. While bio-imaging has nevertheless seen adequate advancement on par to its pharmaceutical counterpart, bio-imaging has been elevated to perform imaging enhancement, in techniques such as MRI [55–57], ultrasound [58–61], *in-vitro* cell imaging [15, 17, 20], and also develop the technologies of imaging as seen in advancement of AFM [4, 21], TEM [22–24], NSOM, and ESEM.

7.4   SCREENSHOT OF REALITY: BIONANO-UNBIASED/UNCENSORED

As seen in detail earlier in *Chapter 6*, we realize that nanotechnology or rather bionanotech has its own limitations in applications and harms the human body, the environment, and the society as a whole. For instance, the toxicity of several nano-particles such as CNT, titania, etc. could cause harm to the body, while nano-metallic particles could pollute the water table and the environment [45]. Having seen the ability of nano-entities of bionanotech to cause harm, it is the need of the hour to set limitations, policies, and regulations to check any possible nano-threat in the near and far future. The need to explore and articulate the toxicology aspects of risk known/unknown nano-entities is reiterated time and again.

Bionanotech needs to be discussed in a public forum, within an industry in small and on a global platform at large [45]. Such a public-discussion would bring into close quarters the opinions of various sections of the society. It is important to know the interests of individuals/industries of varied background and then promote a public opinion based on later decisions. This would help promote a steady and trustable progress in bionano research. A forum that encourages the involvement of participants and non-participants of bionano research will lead to taking into account all ideas, also this will promote to set apt future targets while receiving criticism for the current progress and later goals. The need for the larger role of Federal agencies, public and private industries, environmentalists, law makers, Congress men, Scientists, Physicians, Engineers, and media has been identified. The future of bionano research will depend upon the perspectives of the above-entioned personnel, which could be quite different from one another.

Creating public awareness about the present and future of bionano research and investments will promote healthy participation of the informed-masses. However, to realize such participation adequate research needs to be done in social, economic, ethical, and toxic aspects of bionano industries. This would translate into setting up of newer boundaries, framed-policies, regulations, safety-handling, waste treatment, and safe-disposal of bionano products, for the future [45]. With the present progress and short—comings in mind, there have been predictions about how nanotechnology, including bionanotechnology will impact the near and far future, which can be referred elsewhere [62]. In the following section, we present a roadmap to the realization of translational research in bionanotechnology. Much of the roadmap is about the developments in the global nano-leaders, their initiatives, and the associated funding scenario.

7.5   THE NANO MISSION: ROADMAP TO REALIZATION OF TRANSLATION RESEARCH

Having taken into consideration every aspect of success and failure, advantages and disadvantages, gain and harm, the government, private industries, academia, scientists, and other participants have carefully planned their investments in the form of funds, time, material, and other resources to be allocated for future bionano research. An overall surveillance of the scenario indicates an overwhelming support and trust from various levels of participation in research. In this section, we present the current and future budgets of world leaders in bionanotech. An assessment of the global interest in bionano indicates the keen inclination of various countries to participate and compete in the "nano-race." Currently, there is a steady progress in bionano research. Also there is enough planning and preparatory ground-work to participate in the global competition. The nanomission is to realize the nano-visions and is substantially backed up with adequate interest, directions, resources, funding, planning knowledge, facts, and initiative.

THE BIONANO OUTLOOK: A GLOBAL UPDATE

7.5.1   Bionano in the US

The National Nanotechnology Initiative (NNI) formulated and devised in 2001 by the then American President Bill Clinton [63]. Having attained Federal status and importance the NNI has grown into newer heights in the Bush's administration [63]. Year 2003 is to be marked in history for having made the NNI's mission into a Public Law: 108–153, referred to as

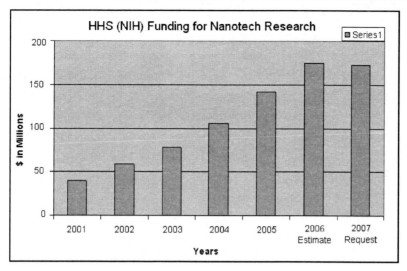

FIGURE 7.1: NNI budget for NIH–HHS granted for bionanotechnology research

"21st Century Nanotechnology Research and Development Act" [63]. The efforts and mission of NNI have been well augmented by Federal funding and National efforts in grooming-up the R&D work. NNI has received global recognition and plays a larger role in determining the future of bionanotechnology. Bionano could be classified under various sections of the 13 Federal Agencies involved in NNI. The most important of all the agencies is the National Institute of Health (NIH), head-quartered at Bethesda, Maryland [28]. The NIH funding received from NNI is shown in Fig. 7.1; it shows a brief history of how the funding has increased in the past few years [48, 64].

The NNI funding "emphasizes on nanotechnology-based biomedical advances occurring at the intersection of biology and the physical sciences" [48]. Moreover, the funding for the department of Health and Human Services (HHS) is mainly utilized for NIH and National Institute of Occupational Safety and Health (NIOSH). A brief look into the tune of monetary support allocated to HHS highlights the promising future of bionanotechnology. The following graph indicates the Federal funding for HHS, of which NIH shares a larger portion. State level supported academic institutions' pioneering research in bionanotechnology includes Stanford University, UPenn, the University of Wisconsin-Madison, Purdue, GATech, Caltech, Drexel University, and many more.

Other global competitors in bionanotechnology include, but not limited to UK, Japan, and the EU. In the following section, we present the initiatives of UK, Japan, and the EU in developing bionanotechnology.

7.5.2 Bio-Nano in Japan

Japan, the second largest economy in the world, is one of the world leaders in nanotechnology not far behind the United States. Since early years, Japan has been an able global competitor in nanotechnology. The National funding and research in the nano realm is carried out directly under the guidance of relevant Japanese ministries [65, 66]. The Japanese interest in bionanotechnology is seen in the form of nanotechnology initiatives in medicine, biotechnology and nano-materials, to the tune of 23 billion Yen, as early as 2001 [65]. The initiative by the Japanese government to keep-up the pace in the international bio-nano race is quite evident from the orchestrated ideology of Japan to partner with Western counterparts [4, 66].

7.5.3 Bio-Nano in UK

The UK has shown immense interest in research in bionanotechnology; it has formed strategic partnerships with US, Japan, the European Union, etc. to significantly contribute to technological advancement. UK enjoys a close tie-up with the United States in developing bionanotech. The Interdisciplinary Research Collaboration (IRC), set up in 2002, is solely dedicated for bionano applications [12]. UK has also partnered with Korea and Japan in several bionano projects [12, 67], some notable ones include—dynamic imaging by high-speed AFM, signal transduction by solid state NMR, energy conversion by new-generational nano-measurement systems, bionanotechnology systems (bio-motors and chemo-sensory systems), DNA nano structures, advanced fluorescence imaging, single-molecule detection, single-molecule AFM, fighting viruses, novel drug development, etc [12].

The basic idea behind the IRC initiative is *"to learn from nature—to understand the structure and function of biological devices and to utilize Nature's solutions in advancing science and engineering in areas as diverse as biosensors, genomics, the discovery of new medicines, diagnostics, and drug delivery."*

7.5.4 UK–Japan Joint Initiative for Bionanotechnology

The British "Biotechnology and Biological Sciences Research Council" (BBSRC) and the "Japan Science and Technology Agency" (JST) have jointly begun an initiative in promoting bionanotechnology [67]. Lucid plans have been laid forth 2003–2008 in promoting bionanotechnology as one of its foremost interests [4, 67]. The gigantic development in biotechnology and sciences has led forth to further development which can be achieved through nano-means and hence the bionano joint venture blossomed.

7.5.5 The EU Initiative in Bionanotech

In the gearing race for Bionano, the European Union is no exception. The European Union formed the sixth Framework Program (FP6) alliance for ground-breaking research in Science

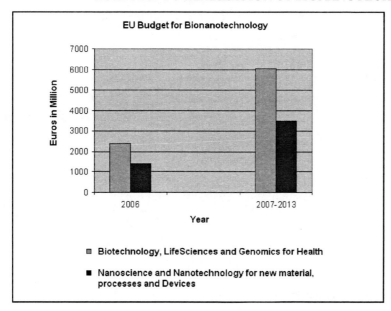

FIGURE 7.2: EU budget for bionanotechnology and associated research

& Technological Advancement [68]. Of the seven thematic priorities identified by EU under the scope of FP6, two are exclusively for biotechnology and nanotechnology which concentrate on [68]:

- Nano-technologies and nano-sciences
- Life sciences, Genomics and Biotechnology for Health

Bionanotechnology claims a substantial portion of the funds allocated for the FP6 research. Fig. 7.2 shows the funds allocated by EU under the Scope of FP6 (2006) and FP7 (2007–13) respectively, for bionanotech associated research. Presently efforts are on the move in creating a roadmap for a smooth transition from FP6 to FP7 (way of the future) which would determine the advancement of science and technology in various applications [69]. The FP7 initiative of the EU corresponds to research during 2007–2013. Of the €50⁺ billions allocated to FP7, about 20% is directly routed to bionanotechnology and its associated research fields such as nano-devices and nano-materials [69].

It is quite evident from the information presented in this chapter that bionano undoubtedly has a promising future as of the preparatory work, funding and access to resource are concerned. However, efforts need to be taken to ensure the same trust, harmony and involvement of various sections/industries/countries of the society/global community is preserved and taken-forth into the future. This requires a larger participation from FDA, NIH, and other federal agencies. It is the duty of the Federal Agencies to guide the research in the right direction. Smaller goals must be set while in transition from the present to future along the roads of development in bionanotechnology. In the words of Richard Feynman *"What would happen if we could arrange atoms one by one the way we want them?"* Hinting at the bottom-up approach on self-assembling techniques, Feynman's world of bionano systems would soon be realized in the near future. As envisioned by Eric Drexler, self-assembling bionano systems—building a nano assembler or a nano surveillance system to perform *in vivo* functions has been a long-standing dream waiting to become true [70]. The day is not far off to realize the nano-visions. In the later section of *this Chapter*, we present you an interesting discussion on the feasibility and future of "molecular assemblers" by Eric Drexler and Richard Smalley.

7.5.6   Bionano in Asia

Asia accounts to 60% of the world population, in which India and China together claim more than one-third (33%) of the total human population. The rapidly growing economy in Asia and its participation in various global competitions cannot be neglected easily. The investment of China and India in bionanotechnology is a result of the booming biotech industries and nanotechnology in both countries. Recently India has signed tie-ups with the United States in nanotechnology research, including bionanotechnology [71]. Here, we present an insight into India's development in bionano research initiatives and progress.

India: The country has plunged itself into deep-waters of bionanotechnology. There has been appreciable development in the past five years in bionano research throughout the nation. India and its research interests are unique in many aspects. Often the diseases and ailments faced by the third-world countries (developing nations) are quite different from that of developed nations, and hence it is of top priority to promote bionano research to address specific issues, common to developing nations. Some worth-while development in Indian bionano research includes [71,72]:

Water purification: Using nano-tubes to filter out viruses as small as 25 nm, e.g., polio virus, E. coli, other pathogens, and bacteria can be filtered out.

Typhoid detection kit: New method to identify S. typhi (typhoid causing) antigen, 30 times more sensitive than present techniques and requires only 2–3 µl serum sample.

Drug delivery: US patented, reverse micelle based "smart" hydrogels for encapsulating water soluble drugs, diameter less than 100 nm.

Medical implants: Developing drug delivery systems for stem cell implants for applications in cardiology, ophthalmology, oncology, endocrinology, etc.

Bionano has greatly impacted India and is being actively pursued not only in Research but also in Industries and Education [73]. Most of the above-mentioned researches are coordinated by the Indian "Nano Science and Technology Consortium" (NASTCON). The major bionano initiatives focus on biotech, biochips, medical, and sensor applications. India is working toward capturing a $50 billion market in the next 10 years, of which bionano (Health Care) is one of the top-priority [72].

The bionano fever has had a great impact on several countries in the East Asian region. Countries such as Singapore, South Korea, Taiwan, Malaysia, etc. are eagerly participating in developing bionano applications. Singapore, for instance, is committed to pursue bionano research in a novel way by bringing in international community to participate in its Bionano initiatives [69,74]. The BioNano International Singapore Pte. Ltd [74] is one such notable initiative from Singapore to promote bionano research. It is a bionanotechnology company dedicated in developing newer bionano-techniques, focusing on developing bionano sensors, bionano-probes, bionano-electrodes, bionano-electro-chemical workstations and bionano-instruments [74].

THE SMALLEY–DREXLER DEBATE: CAN NANOTECHNOLOGY CHANGE THE FUNDAMENTALS OF CHEMISTRY?

Background

Nobel Laureate Richard Errett Smalley and best selling author Kim Eric Drexler are uncrowned gurus of the shrinking world of nanotechnology. Their ground breaking research and phenomenal contributions earned them well-deserved respect in the scientific society. Dr. Smalley (June 6, 1943–October 28, 2005) won the Nobel Prize for Chemistry in 1996 for his invention of C60 or Fullerenes, often referred to as the "Buckyballs". He was the Gene and Norman Hackerman Professor of Chemistry at Rice University, and his pioneering research focused on Carbon Nanotubes [75] and its translation to cancer drug delivery among others. Dr. Drexler is a creative genius and presently the Chief Technical Advisor of Nanorex Inc., involved in the development of computational modeling tools specifically for the design and analysis of productive nanosystems. Dr. Drexler earned one of his PhDs in Molecular Nanotechnology (MNT) from the MIT Media Labs in 1991, the first of its kind ever. Dr. Drexler is presently instrumental in the development of nano ENGINEER 1, 3D nanomechanical CAD software that could be used to design nanosystems [76].

In December 2003, Dr. Drexler and Dr. Smalley argued their points for and against "molecular assemblers", respectively. Dr. Smalley openly criticized the concept of molecular assemblers, envisioned by Dr. Drexler. Their arguments were published by the American Chemical Society's (ACS) journal, Chemical and Engineering News (C&EN), under "POINT and COUNTER-POINT," as a widely cited cover story [77]. In the following section, we present the gist of the for and against arguments on the question: "Are molecular assemblers—devices capable of positioning atoms and molecules for precisely defined reactions in almost any environment—physically possible" [77].

Drexler's phenomenal book, *Engines of Creation: The Coming Era of Nanotechnology*, published in 1986, envisions of a world with molecular assembler, performing precision engineering with almost no pollution. In one of the chapters, "*Engines of Destruction*," the author examines the possibilities of the destructive effects of such molecular assemblers, where he quotes: "Replicating assemblers and thinking machines poses basic threats to people and to life on Earth" [77]. This pioneer in the field of molecular nanotechnology is convinced about the capabilities of molecular assemblers and recognizes the potential risk associated with what he believes they are capable of.

Three books encompass the main ideas of Drexler; *Engines of Creation* was his first book, and later he modified his PhD thesis into a book titled *Nanosystems: Molecular Machinery, Manufacturing and Computation* in 1992, winning him the *Best Computer Science Book of the year—1992* from the Association of American Publishers. The third book was *Unbounding the Future: the Nanotechnology Revolution*. Through his books and journal publications, Drexler presented his visions of a molecular assemblers (nano-factories) that would create nano-factories and nano-machines at a very small scale [77]. He argues that his system of molecular assembler would be like a "robotic arm" controlled by a computer which employs conveyor belts and other nano-machineries to transport the required molecules to the site of interest, and then by the process of "Mechanosynthesis," suitably position the molecules in strategic positions such that a desired reaction is favored [77].

The Feasibility of Molecular Assemblers

Smalley argues that using a computer-controlled arm or a robotic arm could eventually bring together reactants and even bias occurrence of a reaction, but it is not necessarily the desired reaction. Further, Smalley refutes Drexler's argument of seeking an alternate condition for a desired reaction to happen on the basis of the absence of a "medium or liquid." Smalley claims that if two reactants when brought together do not result in a favored (desired) reaction, there is a whole array of reasons explained by Chemistry that allow this to occur [77]. As mentioned before by Drexler, Smalley too maintains the critical need of enzymes or enzyme-like entities participating in the molecular assembly in a self-replicating nanorobot (nanobot). Having assumed the presence of enzymes or ribosomes to participate in molecular assembly of the nanobots, Smalley questions if the nanobots have a cell that produces the required enzymes. If so, how do the nanobot get the required enzyme to the right position? What would be the mechanism of error detection and how is correction and replacement of such enzymes performed? Even further, what is the medium that is going to substitute for water in the reaction, because aqueous-unstable systems cannot be created via the present method of molecular assembly? If there is going to be a replacement medium for water in the nanobot systems, how would dry systems, such as lasers or "ultrafast memory," behave? Finally, Smalley questions the feasibility of controlling atoms with precision owing to the fat finger and sticky finger problem [77].

Fat finger refers to the "imprecision, a molecular assembler would have in selecting and placing an atom to achieve a designed purpose" [78]. *Sticky Finger* refers to the arm of the molecular assembler (or) the nanobot which when engaged in atomic assembly encounters a "sticky" problem such that "the atoms of the manipulator hands will adhere to the atom that is being moved" [79]. In lay man's words, the molecular assembler or the hypothetical self-replicating nanobot is engaged in assembling atoms in a particular fashion to achieve a desired task. The robotic arm or the "finger" engaged in such atomic assembly is too big to be accommodated between individual atoms to control them; there isn't enough room to accommodate all the "fingers" of the nanobot. Similarly the fingers of the nanobots will be engaged with more than one (or) the required atom at a given time, while assembling them, thus proving quite sticky to the surrounding atomic and lacks specificity, precision and selectivity.

Drexler defends his stand on the basis that his concept of "molecular assembler" would employ enzymes at the end of the robotic arm performing the assembling labor, a totally mechanical task. He draws analogy of his system with Feynman's idea of using factories to create smaller factories and produce nanomachines with utmost precision [80, 81]. He talks of the existence of a molecular assembler governed by Systems Engineering principles that transcend traditional chemistry borders. Drexler attributes the working of the molecular assembler to machine-phase chemistry rather than to solution-phase chemistry [77]. As mentioned earlier, the participation of conveyors, positioners, etc. play a crucial role in performing the mechanosynthesis resulting in high precision positional control of the reactants, thereby bringing them together in the right co-ordinates to favor the desired reactions. In case of failure of the desired reaction, Drexler suggests the use of a different condition or environment to perform the task to achieve the desired result. Further he says that the very "positional control naturally avoids most side reactions by preventing unwanted encounters between potential reactants." Drexler claims that "when molecules come together and react, their atoms (being "sticky") stay bonded to neighbors" and hence does not see the need for the *Smalley fingers*. Smalley on the other hand rejects Drexler's visions and arguments on the basis of the fundamental principles of Chemistry. However, Drexler points at the feasibility of developing a "Bottom-up strategy: using self-assembly to build solution-phase molecular machines," then he envisions using this, to acquire positional control of synthesis, and then "leveraging this ability to build systems enabling greater control" [77].

Smalley concludes the arguments saying that one cannot "make precise chemistry occur as desired between two molecular objects with simple mechanical motion along a few degrees of freedom in the assembler-fixed frame of reference" [77]. Such works require guiding reactants through a specific reaction coordinate, lying in a "many-dimensional hyperspace." Creating a "let alone self-replicating assembler—cannot be done simply by pushing two molecular objects together," it demands precision-control, and one needs "some sort of molecular chaperone that can also serve as a catalyst" [77]. All atoms do not freely move when a molecule is moved, there is a plethora of subtle factors cooperating to bring a reaction to completion, unseen and many times misunderstood. The issues of "fat finger" and "sticky finger" need to be resolved, and then the presence or absence of enzyme-like tools and water-like media need to be clarified. According to Smalley, the concept of molecular assembly sounds utopian while it merely scares away people by painting a future with "self-replicating monsters (nanobots) all around us." His message is that the essence of Chemistry has largely been forgotten in this envisioned futuristic engineering marvel and needs to be brought back into focus. Smalley does not acknowledge the threats of Nanotechnology, proposed by Drexler [77].

Epilogue

It is our hope that throughout this book, we have conveyed the ability of bionanotechnology to transcend limits, once never known to have been crossed, and go beyond to improve quality of life and health care. It is our desire to guide the reader to the references cited to understand the concepts further and appreciate the details of the innovative approaches and significant results. Fundamental knowledge gained in bionanotechnology is currently being translated to products and devices that will affect patients immediately and in the near future. Further ahead new discoveries will surprise us again and change the landscape. It is still, however, left to us to wisely use this technology and devise environmentally conscious solutions to benefit the most in the long term. Bionanotechnology is soon evolving into an enabling discipline, powerful enough to realize the dreams of the great nano-visionaries, surprising us and continuously expanding our capabilities.

REFERENCES

[1] V. M. Aponte, D. S. Finch, and D. M. Klaus, Considerations for non-invasive in-flight monitoring of astronaut immune status with potential use of MEMS and NEMS devices. *Life Sci.*, vol. **79**(14), p. 1317, 2006.

[2] G. Kotzar, et al., Evaluation of MEMS materials of construction for implantable medical devices. *Biomaterials*, vol. **23**(13), p. 2737, 2002.

[3] N.-C. Tsai, and C.-Y. Sue, Review of MEMS-based drug delivery and dosing systems. *Sensors Actuators A*, in press, corrected proof.

[4]   I. Choi, et al., In situ observation of biomolecules patterned on a PEG-modified Si surface by scanning probe lithography. *Biomaterials*, vol. **27**(26), p. 4655, 2006.

[5]   M. J. Dalby, et al., Changes in fibroblast morphology in response to nano-columns produced by colloidal lithography. *Biomaterials*, vol. **25**(23), p. 5415, 2004.

[6]   R. Haggenmueller, et al., Aligned single-wall carbon nanotubes in composites by melt processing methods. *Chem. Phys. Lett.*, vol. **330**(3–4), p. 219, 2000.

[7]   P. Nikolaev, et al., Gas-phase catalytic growth of single-walled carbon nanotubes from carbon monoxide. *Chem. Phys. Lett.*, vol. **313**(1–2), p. 91, 1999.

[8]   D. Tomanek, *Carbon Nano Tubes—A time line*. 2001 Sept 7, 2001 [cited; Available from: `http://www.pa.msu.edu/cmp/csc/nanotube.html`.

[9]   M. Zhang, Y. Bando, and K. Wada, Sol-gel template preparation of TiO2 nanotubes and nanorods. *J. Mater. Sci. Lett.*, vol. **20**(2), pp. 167–170, 2001.

[10] Y. Zhang, et al., Synthesis of nano/micro zinc oxide rods and arrays by thermal evaporation approach on cylindrical shape substrate. *J. Phys. Chem. B*, vol. **109**(27), pp. 13091–13093, 2005.

[11] A. L. Stroyuk, V. V. Shvalagin, and S. Y. Kuchmii, Photochemical synthesis and optical properties of binary and ternary metal-semiconductor composites based on zinc oxide nanoparticles. *J. Photochem. Photobiol., A: Chem.*, vol. **173**(2), pp. 185–194, 2005.

[12] 3i, "Nanotechnology—size matters building a successful nanotechnology company," *E.I.U.a.t.I.o. Nanotechnology*, 2002.

[13] M. E. Akerman, et al., Nanocrystal targeting in vivo. *Proc. Natl. Acad. Sci.*, vol. **99**(20), pp. 12617–12621, 2002.

[14] A. P. Alivisatos, Perspectives on the physical chemistry of semiconductor nanocrystals. *J. Phys. Chem.*, vol. **100**(31), pp. 13226–13239, 1996.

[15] R. Bakalova, et al., Quantum dots as photosensitizers? *Nat. Biotech.*, vol. **22**(11), p. 1360, 2004.

[16] M. Brauer, In vivo monitoring of apoptosis. Prog. Neuro-Psychopharmacol. *Biol. Psychiatr.*, vol. **27**(2), p. 323, 2003.

[17] W. C. Chan, et al., Quantum dot bioconjugates for ultrasensitive nonisotopic detection. *Science*, vol. **281**(5385), pp. 2016–2018, 1998.

[18] L. Hirsch, et al., Metal nanoshells. *Ann. Biomed. Eng.*, vol. **34**(1), p. 15, 2006.

[19] O. M. Koo, I. Rubinstein, and H. Onyuksel, Role of nanotechnology in targeted drug delivery and imaging: a concise review. *Nanomed.: Nanotechnol., Biol. Med.*, vol. **1**(3), p. 193, 2005.

[20] A. Smith, et al., Engineering luminescent quantum dots for *in vivo* molecular and cellular imaging. *Ann. Biomed. Eng.*, vol. **34**(1), p. 3, 2006.

[21] F. Barrere, et al., Nano-scale study of the nucleation and growth of calcium phosphate coating on titanium implants. *Biomaterials*, vol. **25**(14), p. 2901, 2004.

[22] Z. L. Dong, et al., TEM and STEM analysis on heat-treated and in vitro plasma-sprayed hydroxyapatite/Ti-6Al-4V composite coatings. *Biomaterials*, vol. **24**(1), p. 97, 2003.

[23] Q. Hu, et al., Preparation and characterization of biodegradable chitosan/hydroxyapatite nanocomposite rods via in situ hybridization: a potential material as internal fixation of bone fracture. *Biomaterials*, vol. **25**(5), p. 779, 2004.

[24] V. M. Rusu, et al., Size-controlled hydroxyapatite nanoparticles as self-organized organic-inorganic composite materials. *Biomaterials*, vol. **26**(26), p. 5414, 2005.

[25] S. L. Goodman, P. A. Sims and R. M. Albrecht, Three-dimensional extracellular matrix textured biomaterials. *Biomaterials*, vol. **17**(21), p. 2087, 1996.

[26] N. Morimoto, et al., Nano-scale surface modification of a segmented polyurethane with a phospholipid polymer. *Biomaterials*, vol. **25**(23), p. 5353, 2004.

[27] A. Thapa, et al., Nano-structured polymers enhance bladder smooth muscle cell function. *Biomaterials*, vol. **24**(17), p. 2915, 2003.

[28] V. J. Chen, L. A. Smith and P. X. Ma, Bone regeneration on computer-designed nano-fibrous scaffolds. *Biomaterials*, vol. **27**(21), p. 3973, 2006.

[29] M. A. Pattison, et al., Three-dimensional, nano-structured PLGA scaffolds for bladder tissue replacement applications. *Biomaterials*, vol. **26**(15), p. 2491, 2005.

[30] K. M. Woo, et al., Nano-fibrous scaffolding promotes osteoblast differentiation and biomineralization. Biomaterials. Vol. **28**(2): pp. 335–43, 2007.

[31] Bethesda, *NIH Roadmap: Nanomedicine.*, 2006.

[32] T. S. Binghe Wang, Richard Soltero., *Drug Delivery: Principles and Applications*. Wiley-Interscience, (462), pp. 57–83, 2005.

[33] L. Brannon-Peppas, and J. O. Blanchette, Nanoparticle and targeted systems for cancer therapy. *Adv. Drug Deliv. Rev.*, vol. **56**(11), pp. 1649–1659, 2004.

[34] D. Bremner, *Drug Delivery: Principles and Applications B. Wang, T. Siahaan and R. Soltero*, Eds., (London, United Kingdom: Chemistry & Industry), p. 24, 2005.

[35] P. Couvreur, et al., Nanotechnologies for drug delivery: Application to cancer and autoimmune diseases. *Prog. Solid State Chem.*, vol. **34**(2–4), pp. 231–235, 2006.

[36] R. Duncan, Nanomedicine gets clinical. *Mater. Today*, vol. **8**(8, Supplement 1), p. 16, 2005.

[37] E. Diederichs, J. and R. H. Muller, *Future Strategies for Drug Delivery with Particulate Systems*. (Stuttgart-Germany: Medpharm GmbH Scientific Publishers), pp. 29–45, 1998.

[38] T.M. Fahmy, et al., Targeted for drug delivery. *Mater. Today*, vol. **8**(8, Supplement 1), pp. 18–26, 2005.

[39] P. H. M. Hoet, I. Brueske-Hohlfeld, and O. V. Salata, Nanoparticles-known and unknown health risks. *J. Nanobiotechnol.*, vol. **2**, 2004, pp. given.

[40] M. A. Horton, and A. Khan, Medical nanotechnology in the UK: a perspective from the London centre for nanotechnology. *Nanomedicine*, vol. **2**(1), pp. 42–48, 2006.

[41] S. K. Sahoo, and V. Labhasetwar, Nanotech approaches to drug delivery and imaging. *Drug Discovery Today*, vol. **8**(24), pp. 1112–1120, 2003.

[42] T. Vo-Dinh, P. Kasili, and M. Wabuyele, Nanoprobes and nanobiosensors for monitoring and imaging individual living cells. *Nanomedicine*, vol. **2**(1), pp. 22–30, 2006.

[43] P. D. Vogel, Nature's design of nanomotors. *Eur. J. Pharm. Biopharm.*, vol. **60**(2), pp. 267–277, 2005.

[44] A. Wickline Samuel, and M. Lanza Gregory, Nanotechnology for molecular imaging and targeted therapy. *Circulation*, vol. **107**(8), pp. 1092–5, 2003.

[45] T. R. S.-B. Govt, The Royal Society Report—'Nanoscience and nanotechnologies: opportunities and uncertainties'. *Nanosci. Nanotechnol.*, pp. 1–111, 2004.

[46] V. E. Kagan, H. Bayir, and A. A. Shvedova, Nanomedicine and nanotoxicology: two sides of the same coin. *Nanomed: Nanotechnol., Biol. Med.*, vol. **1**(4), p. 313, 2005.

[47] J. Muller, et al., Respiratory toxicity of multi-wall carbon nanotubes. *Toxicol. Appl. Pharmacol.*, vol. **207**(3), p. 221, 2005.

[48] J. S. M. Tsuji, D. Andrew Howard, Paul C. James, John T. Lam, Chiu-wing Warheit, David B. Santamaria, Annette B., Research strategies for safety evaluation of nanomaterials, part IV: risk assessment of nanoparticles. *Toxicol. Sci.*, vol. **89**(1), pp. 42–50, 2006.

[49] D.B. Warheit, et al., Comparative pulmonary toxicity assessment of single-wall carbon nanotubes in rats. *Toxicol. Sci.*, vol. **77**(1), pp. 117–125, 2004.

[50] M. Ferrari, Cancer nanotechnology: opportunities and challenges. *Nat. Rev. Cancer*, vol. **5**(3), p. 161, 2005.

[51] M. J. Roberts, M. D. Bentley, and J. M. Harris, Chemistry for peptide and protein PEGylation. *Adv. Drug Deliv. Rev.*, vol. **54**(4), p. 459, 2002.

[52] F. Chellat, et al., Therapeutic potential of nanoparticulate systems for macrophage targeting. *Biomaterials*, vol. **26**(35), pp. 7260–7275, 2005.

[53] A. Nagayasu, K. Uchiyama, and H. Kiwada, The size of liposomes: a factor which affects their targeting efficiency to tumors and therapeutic activity of liposomal antitumor drugs. *Adv. Drug Deliv. Rev.*, vol. **40**(1–2), p. 75, 1999.

[54] L. S. A. B. C. Yu, *Dekker Pharmaceutical technology: Biopharmaceutics*. 2002.

[55] D. Thorek, et al., Superparamagnetic Iron Oxide Nanoparticle Probes for Molecular Imaging. *Ann. Biomed. Eng.*, vol. **34**(1), p. 23, 2006.

[56] J. M. Perez, et al., Magnetic relaxation switches capable of sensing molecular interactions. *Nat. Biotech.*, vol. **20**(8), p. 816, 2002.

[57] A. Tanimoto, and S. Kuribayashi, Application of superparamagnetic iron oxide to imaging of hepatocellular carcinoma. *Eur. J. Radiol.*, vol. **58**(2), p. 200, 2006.

[58] F. Calliada, et al., Ultrasound contrast agents: basic principles. *Eur. J. Radiol.*, vol. **27**(Supplement 2), p. S157, 1998.

[59] R. Campani, et al., Contrast enhancing agents in ultrasonography: Clinical applications. *Eur. J. Radiol.*, vol. **27**(Supplement 2), p. S161, 1998.

[60] G. Maresca, et al., New prospects for ultrasound contrast agents. *Eur. J. Radiol.*, vol. **27**(Supplement 2), p. S171, 1998.

[61] B. E. Oeffinger, and M. A. Wheatley, Development and characterization of a nano-scale contrast agent. *Ultrasonics*, vol. **42**(1–9), p. 343, 2004.

[62] J. C. Glenn, *Nanotechnology: future military environmental health considerations B.* Technological Forecast. Social Change, vol. **73**: p. 128–137, 2006.

[63] *History of the National Nanotechnology Initiative (NNI).* 2006 [cited; Available from: http://www.nano.gov/html/about/history.html.

[64] NNI, *National Nanotechnology Initiative (NNI), Research and Development Leading to a Revolution in Technology and Industry, Supplement to President's FY 2006 Budget, March 2005.* 2005.

[65] T. K. A. Y. Bando, Status and trends of nanotechnology R&D in Japan. *Nat. Mater.*, vol. **3**(March), pp. 129–131, 2004.

[66] *Nanotechnology (including bionanotechnology) R&D initiatives in Japan.* 2006 [cited; Available from: http://www.globalwatchservice.com/pages/ThreeColumns. aspx?PageID=146.

[67] *Biotechnology and Biological Sciences Research Council (BBSRC) Report: World Class Bioscience—Strategic Plan 2003–2008.* Updated, British BBSRC. p. 1–47, 2005.

[68] *EU Budget for FP6—Bionanotechnology Research initiative 2006.* 2006 [cited; Available from: http://cordis.europa.eu/fp6/budget.htm.

[69] *EU Funding for FP7, Road Map for FP6 to FP7 (Science and Technology Research Initiatives)—2007 to 2013.* 2006 [cited; Available from: http://cordis.europa.eu/fp7/budget.htm.

[70] S. Goodsell, D., *Bionanotechnology: Lessons from Nature.* John Wiley and Sons Inc. (311), pp. 295–311, 2004.

[71] NASTCON. *Nano Science and Technology Consortium (NASTCON).* 2005 [cited; Available from: http://www.nstc.in/NSTCHead/Research_Area.aspx.

[72]   D. A. P. J. A. Kalam, *President's Address at the Inauguration of the Indo-Us Nanotechnology Conclave*, P.I.B.P.G.o. India, Editor. Wednesday, February 22, 2006, President's Secretariat Govt of India.

[73]   D. Richard, E. B. Booker, *Nanotechnology For Dummies.* pp. 1–384, 2005.

[74]   BioNano. *BioNano International Singapore Pte. Ltd.* 2005 [cited; Available from: http://www.bionano.com.sg/products.htm.

[75]   R. Smalley, *Research Areas of Dr.Smalley.* 2005 [cited 2006; Available from: http://smalley.rice.edu/smalley.cfm?doc_id=4858.

[76]   M. Sims, *Eric Drexler Joins Nanorex.* 2005 [cited 2006; Available from: http://www.nanoengineer-1.com/mambo/index.php?option=com_content&task=view&id=69&Itemid=73.

[77]   R. Baum, Nanotechnology: Drexler and Smalley make the case for and against "molecular assemblers". *Chem. Eng. News*, vol. **81**(48), pp. 37–42, 2003.

[78]   *Fat Fingers.* 2006 [cited; Available from: http://www.nanotitan.com/nCyclopedia/fatFingers.htm.

[79]   R. E. Smalley, Of chemistry, love and nanobots. *Sci. Am.*, vol. **285**(3), pp. 76–77, 2001.

[80]   R. P. Feynman, *There's plenty of room at the bottom.* 1959 [cited; Available from: http://www.zyvex.com/nanotech/feynman.html.

[81]   R. P. Feynman, *Plenty of Room at the Bottom [Courtesy of The Archives, California Institute of Technology].* 1959.

Author Biography

Aravind Parthasarathy earned his Masters Degree from Drexel University in Biomedical Engineering, in 2006. He is presently working as a Product Engineer at EPMedsystems, NJ where he is involved in the design and development of diagnostic equipments for Cardiac Electrophysiology. His research at Drexel concentrated on the applications of Bionanotechnology in health care, and in improvising cardiac pacemakers. He earned his Bachelors degree in Electrical & Electronics Engineering from Bharathidasan University, India. Apart from his writing interests, he does quite a bit of circuit building for applications including medical devices, robotics and controls & instrumentation. He is passionate about realizing his dream of making a nanotechnology based "wireless cardiac pacemaker" and believes in seeing more of nanotech based commercial medical devices in the near future.

Dr. Elisabeth S. Papazoglou is the author of more than 40 original articles and 12 patents in materials and nanotechnology. During her 14 years experience in the chemical industry (Arco Chemical, FMC, Great Lakes) she led basic and applied R&D and developed novel commercial products based on nanotechnology. Dr. Papazoglou holds a Diploma in Chemical Engineering from the Aristotelian University of Thessaloniki, Greece, a Masters in Chemical Engineering from the University of Delaware and a Ph.D. in Macromolecular Science & Polymer Engineering from Case Western Reserve University. She is currently an Assistant Professor in the School of Biomedical Engineering at Drexel University where her research focuses on Bionanotechnology especially on the unique properties of nanoparticles for simultaneous delivery and imaging applications. Her expertise includes, but is not limited to nano approach in wound healing, nano imaging of skin chemistry and QDs based study of skin inflammation.